Self-assessment picture tests
Oral
Diseas

P-J Lamey
BSc BDS MBChB DDS FDS
RCPS FFD RCSI

Professor of Oral Medicine
School of Clinical Dentistry
The Queen's University of Belfast
Belfast, UK

W H Binnie
DDS MSD FRCPath

Professor of Oral Pathology
Baylor College of Dentistry
Dallas, Texas, USA

R H Johnson
DDS MSD

Professor of Periodontics
School of Dentistry
University of Washington
Seattle, Washington, USA

D G MacDonald
RD* ADC BDS PhD FRCPath
FDS RCPS

Professor of Oral Pathology
Glasgow Dental Hospital and School
Glasgow, UK

M Mosby-Wolfe

London • Baltimore • Barcelona • Bogotá • Boston
Buenos Aires • Carlsbad, CA • Chicago • Madrid
Mexico City • Milan • Naples, FL • New York
Philadelphia • St Louis • Seoul • Singapore
Sydney • Taipei • Tokyo • Toronto • Wiesbaden

Publisher:	**Geoff Greenwood**
Development Editor:	**Simon Pritchard**
Project Manager:	**Dave Burin**
Production:	**Siobhan Egan**
Cover Design:	**Lara Last**
Index:	**Nina Boyd**

Copyright © 1997 Times Mirror International Publishers Limited

Published in 1997 by Mosby-Wolfe, an imprint of Times Mirror International Publishers Limited

Printed in Italy by Vicenzo Bona s.r.l., Turin

ISBN 0 7234 2397 0

For full details of all Times Mirror International Publishers Limited titles, please write to Times Mirror International Publishers Limited, Lynton House, 7–12 Tavistock Square, London WC1H 9LB, England.

A CIP catalogue record for this book is available from the British Library.

PREFACE

This book is a culmination of many years of experience in the specialties of oral medicine and oral pathology. The authors have collaborated jointly in selecting clinical cases, many of which have an oral pathology component. Both rare and common diseases have been chosen to provide a comprehensive spectrum of oro-facial disease.

The intended audience are final year dental and medical students and post-graduates, including those preparing for higher qualifications. Each clinical case poses several questions of varying difficulty selected for the diagnostic and management problems they pose. Although a book of this size cannot be encyclopedic, it does test a broad base of clinico-pathological knowledge. Like all learning experiences it is also meant to be enjoyable.

P-J Lamey

W H Binnie

R H Johnson

D G MacDonald

ACKNOWLEDGEMENT

We would like to express our thanks and gratitude to Mrs Theresa McNally for providing all the secretarial support.

QUESTIONS

QUESTIONS

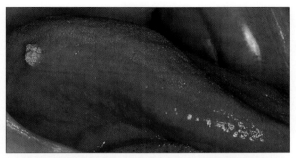

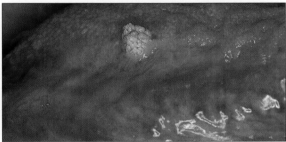

▲ 1 An edentulous 53-year-old man noticed a small growth on his tongue, which had been present for at least 2 years. The growth was symptom free and had not changed in size during that period.

Except for chronic bronchitis, his medical history was essentially normal. He was married, unemployed, an occasional pipe smoker and a social drinker.

Clinical examination revealed a vegetative growth, 5 mm in diameter, on the right lateral border of the tongue. The lesion was excised.

(a) What is the likely diagnosis?
(b) What clinical features suggest an infective origin?
(c) What is the multiple variant of the disease called?
(d) What is responsible for these lesions?
(e) The lateral margin of the tongue is a frequent site of malignancy. Is this lesion malignant or potentially so?

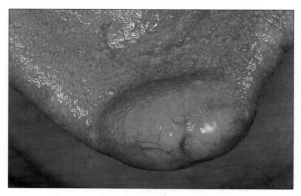

▲ 2 A 48-year-old woman who was referred with
bilateral white patches on the buccal mucosa. The
patient was a suspected late-onset diabetic on no
medication. She had been in hospital for a varicose vein
operation and was taking atenolol for hypertension and
analgesics.

The patient was single, drank alcohol only
occasionally and did not smoke. She had had her teeth
extracted 12 years ago and once complete dentures had
been inserted she had not returned to the dentist.

On examination white patches were noted on the
right and left buccal mucosae, lateral borders and
dorsal surface of the tongue, and floor of the mouth.
There also was a large firm swelling on the tip of the
tongue, about 20 mm in diameter. An incisional biopsy
of the right buccal mucosa and an excisional biopsy of
the lingual swelling were performed.
(a) What name is given to the triad of lichen planus,
diabetes and essential hypertension?
(b) What is the possible role of drug therapy in this
case?
(c) What is the differential diagnosis for the tongue
lesion?

▶ **3** An 11-year-old girl was referred by her general dental practitioner regarding a swelling on the gingiva labial to the overlying central incisor. The lesion had been present for approximately 1 year and the child

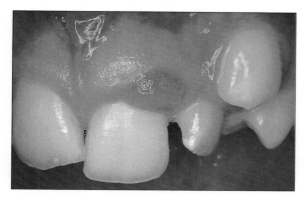

was scheduled to begin orthodontic therapy.

Medical history revealed that the girl suffered from asthma and used a hydrocortisone cream to control eczema.

A relatively firm lesion at the gingival margin of the maxillary left central incisor was detected on clinical examination. A provisional diagnosis of pyogenic granuloma was made and an excisional biopsy was performed.
(a) Give three differential diagnoses.
(b) Is steroid cover required before biopsy?

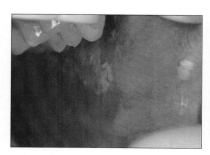
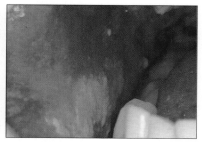

▲ **4** This 8-year-old girl was referred by her doctor for what was described as chronic thrush. The condition was noted at birth and had failed to respond to long-term topical antifungal drugs. Otherwise the child was entirely healthy. The lesions were bilateral and her father had similar but less clinically obvious lesions.
(a) List four differential diagnoses.
(b) What is the most likely diagnosis?
(c) How does this condition arise?
(d) What other body sites may be involved?

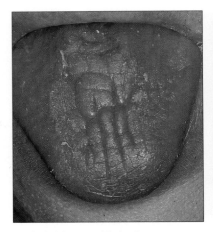 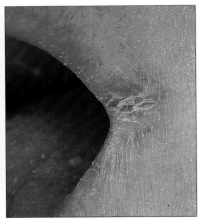

▲ **5** A 44-year-old single woman attended the Oral Medicine Clinic as an emergency patient with the complaint that 'her gums feel poisoned and her mouth feels dry'. Her social and medical history was complex. She had been hospitalised for two minor cerebrovascular accidents, termination of pregnancies, 14 attempted drug overdoses and an unsuccessful suicide from a bridge. The patient was buying diazepam from a neighbour because her family doctor would not give her a prescription. She had been an alcoholic for 8 years and her male partner was physically abusing her. She was attending a psychiatrist. She did not smoke.

Clinical examination revealed angular cheilitis with xerostomia. Routine haematological and microbiological investigations were conducted. A moderate growth of *Candida albicans* was discovered on an oral rinse. The levels of antinuclear antibody and rheumatoid factor were measured and found to be positive at a titre of 1:128.

(a) Is chronic anxiety or depression likely to produce this degree of xerostomia?

(b) Is diazepam abuse likely to produce xerostomia?

(c) Is chronic alcoholism likely to produce xerostomia?

(d) Is the isolation of significant numbers of candidal species intraorally to be expected?

(e) What is the biopsy of choice to investigate her xerostomia and what precautions would need to be taken in this case?

(f) What is rheumatoid factor and with what diseases is it associated?

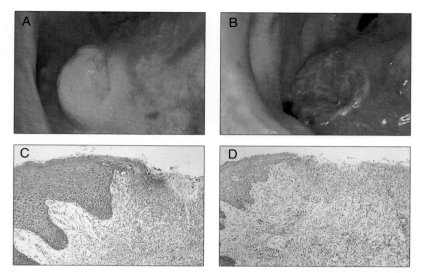

▲ 6 The patient was a 72-year-old retired woman whose chief complaint was
a large, painful ulcer of 3 weeks' duration on the right side of her tongue.
Two years earlier she had visited the clinic because of suspected aphthous
ulceration and underwent full blood screening, which showed no
abnormality. She suffered from osteoarthritis and had been hospitalised for
the treatment of cardiac arrhythmias. The patient took an antiarrythmic drug
and purchased analgesics daily. She stopped smoking cigarettes (under 10 per
day) 2 years previously, but did drink four whiskies a week. Her current set of
complete dentures were a few months old. An initial incisional biopsy was
obtained. One week later, the lesion was subject to excisional biopsy.

(a) At this site what lesion has to be excluded?
(b) Describe the histological features of the first biopsy (C).
(c) Why was the biopsy repeated?
(d) Describe the histological features of the second biopsy (D).
(e) Following the second biopsy, healing was uneventful. How would you
manage the patient subsequently?

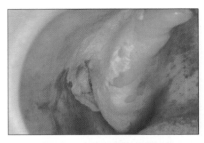

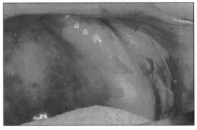

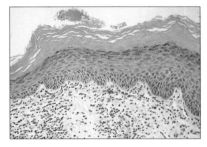

◀ 7 This patient's initial visit to the Oral Medicine Clinic occurred 5 years ago. At that time she was 63 years old, smoked 15 cigarettes per day and drank alcohol socially. She had been referred because of extensive white patches on the maxillary alveolar ridge under a complete denture. Routine haematological investigations revealed a ferritin level of 10 ng/ml (normal range 25–300 ng/ml). Microbiological results were essentially normal. The patient refused to have the white patches biopsied. Five years later the patient returned. She had no apparent medical problems but still smoked 10 cigarettes a day. Photographs of the leukoplakic areas were taken and permission for an incisional biopsy was given.
(a) Should the patient be prescribed iron therapy?
(b) What effect does iron have on the oral epithelium?
(c) Comment on the histological features.
(d) Outline the main steps in management.

▲ 8 (a) Name two ocular complications of mucous membrane pemphigoid.
(b) What respiratory infection can be reactivated by long-term, high-dose corticosteroids?
(c) Why was pemphigus previously fatal?

9 List three benefits of acyclovir cream in treating herpes labialis.

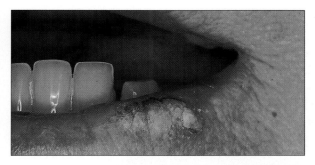

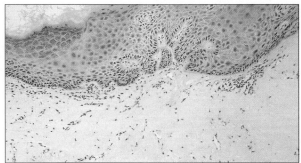

▲ **10** A 71-year-old retired gentleman was referred because of a crusting on his lower lip of 15 years' duration that recently had increased in size. He suffered from a mild cerebrovascular accident 3 years ago, which had left him with a slight speech defect. He had undergone cataract surgery and stopped smoking cigars 5 years ago.

On clinical examination a slightly raised, rough asymptomatic lesion (10 × 6 mm in size) was noted on the left side of the patient's lower lip. Microbiological investigation revealed no growth of candidal organisms. An incision biopsy was performed.

At the routine 3-month review the lesion was still present and the patient was concerned about its appearance. He was referred for surgical excision of the lesion.

(a) What are the two differential diagnoses?
(b) What are the main histological features evident?
(c) Should the patient be asked about his previous occupation?

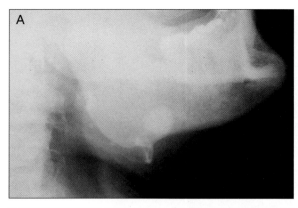

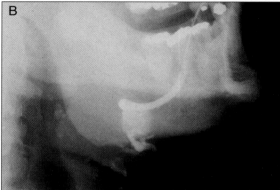

◀ **11** This healthy 28-year-old man complained of recurrent swelling in the submandibular region for 4 months. The swelling could arise at mealtimes but arose at other times as well. The swelling, which was clinically visible, subsided entirely in about half an hour.
(a) What does the plain radiograph **A** show?
(b) What does the other radiograph **B** show?
(c) Would scintiscanning be helpful?
(d) How would you manage this case?

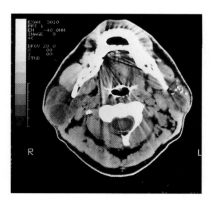

◀ **12** A 40-year-old patient had been diagnosed as HIV positive 4 years earlier. In the previous 4 months he had noted progressive painless enlargement of both parotid glands.
(a) What investigation is being undertaken?
(b) What additional investigation has been undertaken on the left side?
(c) What patholosis is noted?
(d) How would you treat this condition?

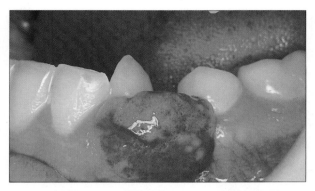

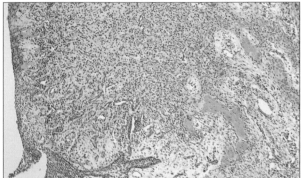

▲ **13** This 16-year-old schoolboy was referred by his dentist complaining of a swelling in the lower left anterior region that had been present for about 6 months and which had, in his own words, 'become infected' in the past 3 months.

The boy's medical history revealed only allergy to grass pollen and animal dander. On clinical examination a large soft swelling of the gingivae in the canine region was noted. An excisional biopsy was performed after radiographs were taken.

(a) Why were radiographs taken?

(b) Give three differential diagnoses.

(c) By 'become infected' the patient meant that the lesion was occasionally painful. What clinical changes account for this?

(d) Describe the histological features and suggest a diagnosis.

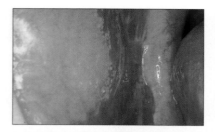

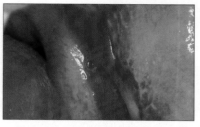

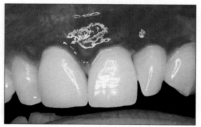

◀ **14** A 49-year-old housewife was referred by her general practitioner. She had been complaining of oral discomfort for many years but this sensation had worsened over the past 6 months. She was a non-smoker and non-drinker and her medical history was clear. On examination she had apparent lichen planus on the right and left buccal mucosa and the dorsum of the tongue and also desquamative gingivitis. A provisional diagnosis of erosive lichen planus and desquamative gingivitis was made. Routine blood and microbiological tests were within the normal range. An incisional biopsy of the left margin of the tongue was undertaken.

(a) What systemic drug therapy could be used to treat this condition?
(b) How many forms of the disease on average do oral lichen planus patients have?
(c) Would systemic drug therapy resolve the desquamative gingivitis?

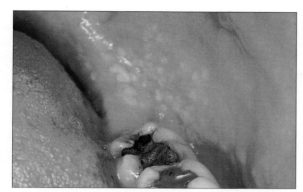

◀ 15 (a) What is the condition?
(b) Is it potentially malignant?
(c) Are these the pathological features expected?

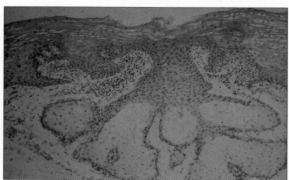

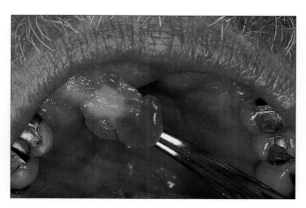

◀ 16 (a) What is this condition?
(b) Is the patient likely to wear a partial denture?
(c) What two management options are appropriate?

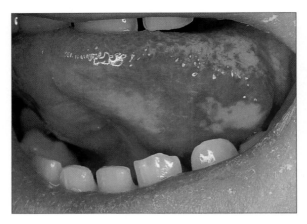

◀ **17** (a) What is responsible for the colour of the base of this ulcer?
(b) What proportion of aphthous ulcers are major in type?
(c) Given that aphthae are not caused by infection, what group of drugs is useful in the treatment of major aphthae?

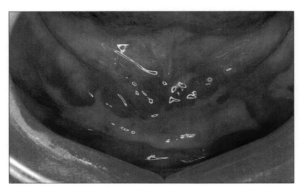

◀ **18** This vesiculobullous condition is relatively painless.
(a) What is the likely diagnosis?
(b) Name three drugs used in its treatment.
(c) Is the condition lifelong?

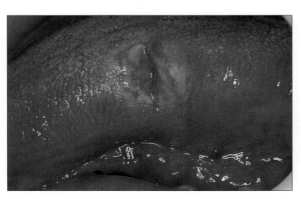

◀ **19** (a) What feature of this lesion suggests the diagnosis?
(b) Are blood tests appropriate?
(c) To what medical speciality should this patient be referred?

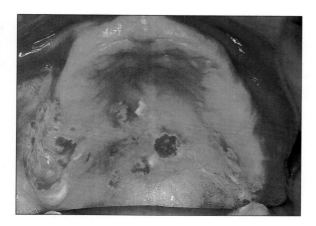

◄ **20** Suggest three diagnoses for this condition.

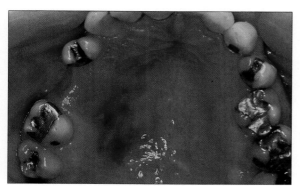

◄ **21** (a) What is this condition?
(b) Is it malignant?
(c) The patient is aged 30 years, so what is the most likely underlying disease?

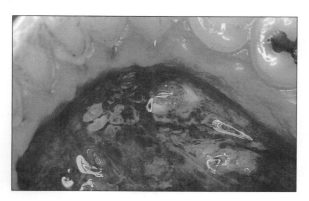

◄ **22** (a) This patient is aged 26 years – does this exclude oral cancer?
(b) Are retinoids effective treatment?
(c) How should such patients be monitored?

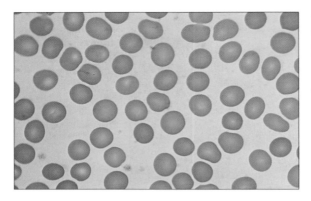

◀ **23** (a) What are these cells?
(b) What stain has been used?
(c) Are they normal?

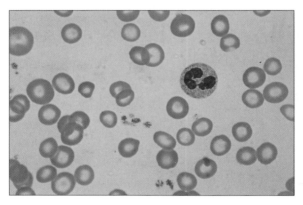

◀ **24** (a) What two cell types are shown?
(b) What abnormality is shown?
(c) What condition does this represent?

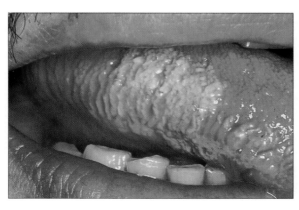

◀ **25** (a) What is this condition?
(b) What is its cause?
(c) What treatment is available?

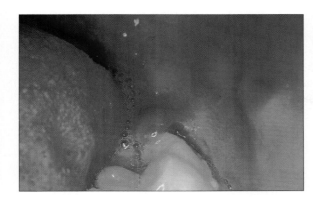

◀ **26** (a) What is this condition? (b) Why did the clinical presentation suggest HIV infection?

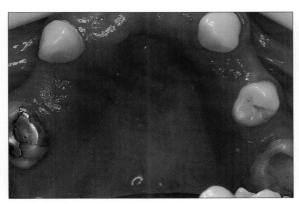

◀ **27** (a) Would you expect to isolate *Candida* from this lesion? (b) Why does it appear red?

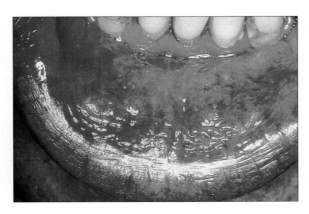

◀ **28** This patient has ulcerative colitis. What are these lesions called?

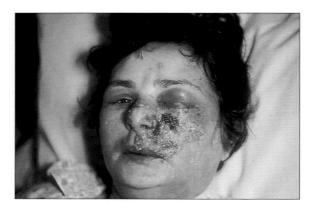

◀ **29** (a) What is this condition?
(b) How should it be treated?
(c) What sequelae may develop?

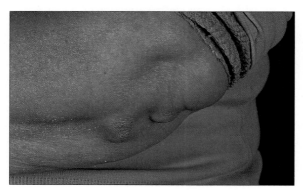

◀ **30** (a) What are these?
(b) To what salivary disease can they be related?

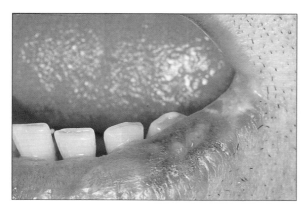

◀ **31** (a) What is this condition?
(b) Is it difficult to treat successfully?
(c) Is it potentially malignant?

▶ 32 A 13-year-old Pakistani boy presented because of a painless swelling palatal to his central incisors. The lesion had been present for about 2 months and apparently was increasing in size. The boy's medical history was unremarkable. He

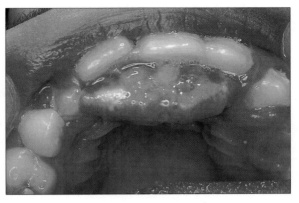

was an irregular dental attender. Examination revealed a large pedunculated firm swelling on the anterior hard palate behind the central incisors. The surface of the swelling was ulcerated and oral hygiene was poor, with generalised plaque and marginal gingivitis.

An excisional biopsy was performed but the lesion recurred three times at the same site over an 18-month period. Significant bone loss had occurred on the palatal aspect of the central incisors.

(a) Suggest four differential diagnoses.
(b) What is the likely diagnosis?
(c) What role may the occlusion play in the development of this lesion?
(d) Why did the lesion recur?
(e) Why was there radiographic evidence of bone loss?

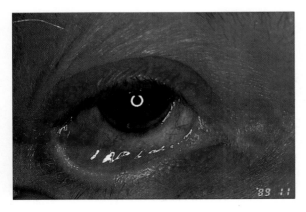

◀ 33 (a) What is wrong with this eye?
(b) With what oral condition is it associated?

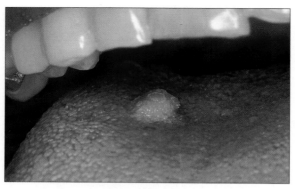

▲ **34** A 67-year-old housewife was referred because of
a lump that she had discovered on her tongue 1 week
previously. The patient was an insulin-dependent
diabetic who smoked three or four cigarettes a day and
drank alcohol socially.

On examination her oral mucosa was generally
healthy but on the dorsum of the tongue there was a
pedunculated growth, which her dental practitioner
thought was a squamous cell papilloma. The lesion was
excised.

(a) Is it likely that this lesion arose over a 1-week
period?

(b) Why is this lesion not a squamous cell papilloma?

(c) What time of day would you choose to excise this
lesion under local anaesthesia?

(d) What is the differential diagnosis?

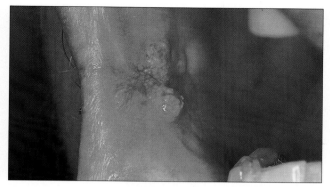

▲ **35** (a) Is this a squamous cell papilloma and if not, why not?

(b) Is biopsy indicated?

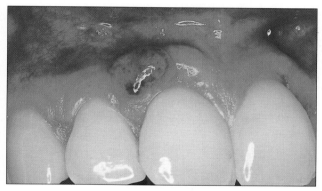

▲ **36** A 42-year-old healthy, non-smoking and non-drinking, married woman was referred by her general medical practitioner because of a painless swelling on the gingiva adjacent to the maxillary right central incisor.

Examination showed an erythematous swelling on the attached gingiva distolabial of the maxillary right central incisor. Radiographs revealed no pathosis. A series of blood tests was performed; the only abnormality was a low ferritin level. The lesion was excised.

(a) Is the low ferritin level relevant to this condition?

(b) What are the main differential diagnoses?

(c) Are any other blood tests indicated?

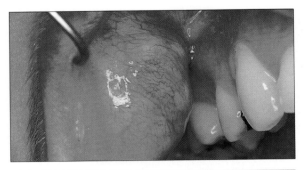

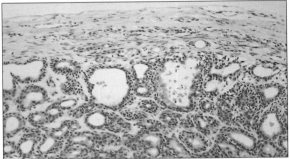

▲ 37 A 37-year-old woman was referred by her
dentist because of a swelling on the inside of her left
cheek, which had been present for several years. The
swelling was painless and showed no recent increase in
size.

An excisional biopsy was performed.
(a) List four differential diagnoses.
(b) What is the likely diagnosis?
(c) Describe the features seen in the photomicrograph.
(d) Based on the microscopic appearance what is the
likely diagnosis?

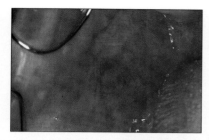

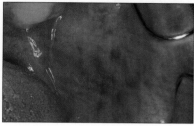

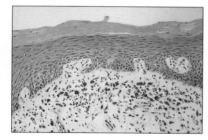

◀ **38** A 46-year-old woman presented complaining of 'bruises' inside her cheeks.

The patient suffered from a back injury for which she took non-steroidal anti-inflammatory drugs and calcium; she was receiving diuretic drugs for hypertension. She smoked 15–20 cigarettes a day. Oral examination revealed diffuse, bluish–grey discoloration on the right and left buccal mucosae. The results of haematological investigations, including electrolytes, were normal and the patient was normotensive. An incisional biopsy of the right buccal mucosa was performed.

(a) What are the main differential diagnoses for the oral findings?

(b) From the history what makes Addison's disease highly unlikely?

(c) Is a platelet count likely to be helpful?

(d) If the patient were HIV positive would that be significant in terms of the oral changes?

(e) What are the main histological features?

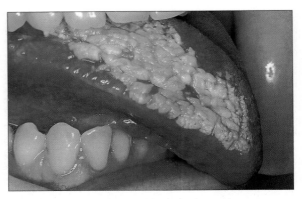

▲ **39** A healthy 36-year-old married woman was
referred by her general practitioner with a 6-year
history of leukoplakia that apparently had been
biopsied when it was first noticed but which had
recurred. A 1-week course of systemic fluconazole had
been prescribed by her general medical practitioner.
The patient had smoked 30 cigarettes a day since the
age of 17 and was a non-drinker.

An extensive leukoplakic patch on the right side of
the dorsum of the tongue was seen on oral
examination. Routine microbiological and
haematological investigations revealed no
abnormalities. An incisional biopsy was performed.

(a) Is the condition likely to be related to her smoking
habit?

(b) What is the significance of the patient's age?

(c) Comment on the likely histological features.

(d) What treatment options are available?

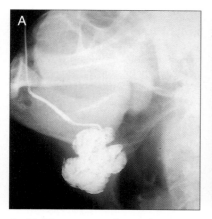 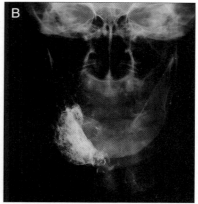

▲ **40** These two radiographs were taken 1 week apart. The patient had a previous history of head and neck irradiation for a lymphoma.
(a) What investigation is being undertaken in (**A**)?
(b) What material has been used to obtain this radiograph and why?
(c) What has happened in the second radiograph (**B**)?
(d) What is the prognosis?

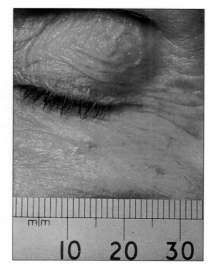

◀ **41** This 70-year-old lady was referred to the Oral Medicine Clinic by her dentist for management of oral candidosis. She was noted to have a lesion below her eye although she herself was unaware of it.
(a) What is the likely diagnosis?
(b) What is the treatment of choice?
(c) Are similar lesions likely to appear on the forehead?

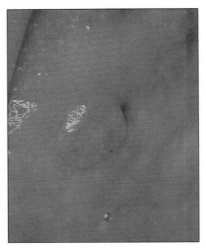

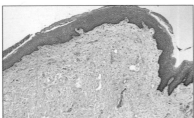

◄ **42** This patient was a 52-year-old gentleman, referred with a small swelling in the right buccal mucosa. His only complaint was that he occasionally bit this.

The medical history revealed nothing of note, except hospitalisation some years previously for chest pains. He was taking no medication, was a non-smoker and drank up to six whiskies per week. He was partially dentate and wore a partial upper denture that he kept in at night. He was an irregular dental attender.

On examination, his palate was found to be erythematous and there was an elevated smooth lesion on the right buccal mucosa. An excisional biopsy was performed and also an oral rinse for microbiological investigation.

(a) Is the buccal mucosal lesion related to his probable erythematous candidiasis of the palate?

(b) What are the main histological features of the excised lesion?

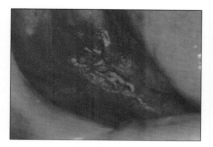 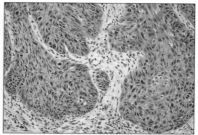

▲ **43** The patient was an 87-year-old woman referred by her general practitioner concerning a white patch in her mouth, which was causing her some pain.

Her medical history revealed an unspecified heart condition for which she was prescribed digoxin and frusemide. She said her mouth had felt swollen for the last 6 months. Her general practitioner had treated the condition with topical nystatin antifungal therapy to no effect.

Clinically the patient had a red and white patch on her lower right edentulous ridge. She also had an erythematous candidiasis beneath her upper complete denture.

Blood tests, including fasting blood glucose, were all normal. The oral rinse showed a heavy growth of *Candida albicans*. An incisional biopsy of the lower alveolar mucosa was performed and the patient placed on fluconazole 50 mg daily for 1 week.

(a) Could the lesion of the lower alveolus be due to candidal infection?
(b) Comment on the histological appearance of the lesion.

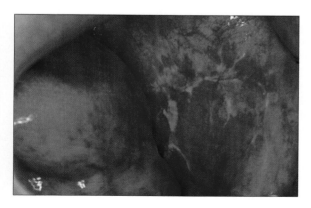

◀ **44** (a) What is this condition?
(b What age group does it affect?
(c) How many forms of the condition are usually present at one time?

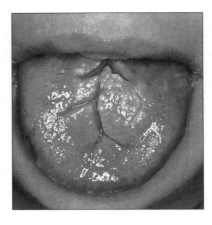

◀ **45** This patient also has chronic nailbed lesions.
(a) What three abnormalities are present?
(b) What is causing the white areas?
(c) What is this group of conditions called?

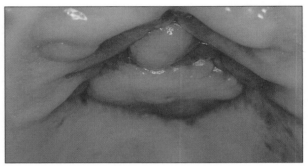

▲ **46** A 55-year-old housewife had been aware of an asymptomatic, slowly growing lesion in the roof of her mouth for at least 10 years. The patient was referred because the lesion was interfering with the fit of her complete upper denture.

Her medical history revealed rheumatoid arthritis and a suspected duodenal ulcer for which she took cimetidine. She smoked 30 cigarettes a day and was a social drinker. On clinical examination a pedunculated fibrous lesion was discovered, which was excised under local anaesthesia.
(a) Does the duration of the lesion exclude malignancy?
(b) Why is the lesion pedunculated?
(c) What is the likely diagnosis?
(d) Is her medical history significant in terms of development of the lesion?

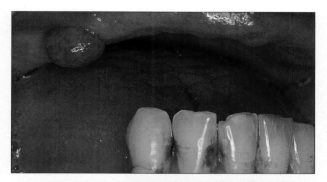

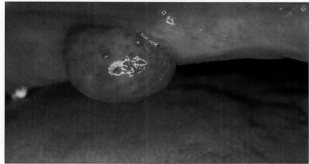

▲ **47** A 57-year-old retired lorry driver was referred by his general dental practitioner regarding a soft tissue swelling on the edentulous ridge in the region of the maxillary right canine. He smoked four cigarettes a week. His medical history revealed that he suffered from angina and emphysema. He used an albuterol inhaler and took co-proxamol and prednisolone.

In addition to the lesion, clinical examination revealed erythematous candidiasis, which was treated with topical antifungal therapy and improved denture hygiene. The lump was excised for microscopic evaluation.

(a) What investigations would be worthwhile preoperatively and why?

(b) What medical treatment should be undertaken prior to biopsy?

(c) Has the patient's drug therapy contributed to the oral candidiasis?

(d) List four differential diagnoses for the soft tissue swelling.

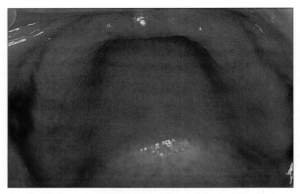

▲ **48** This patient wears complete upper and lower dentures.
(a) What abnormality is seen?
(b) What is this condition called?
(c) Is it painful?
(d) What factors predispose to this condition?

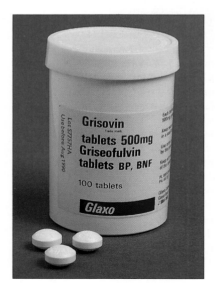

◀ **49** (a) What kind of drug is this?
(b) For what is it normally used?
(c) What oral condition can it be used to treat?

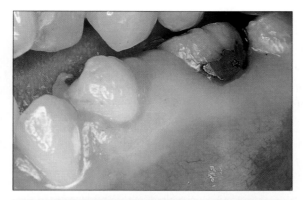

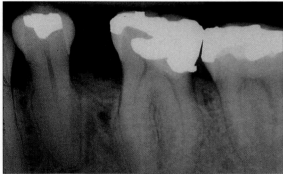

▲ **50** This 29-year-old nursery nurse was referred to the Oral Medicine Clinic because of an asymptomatic, firm swelling in the region of the mandibular left second premolar. The patient was taking ranitidine for a duodenal ulcer and displayed a class III malocclusion. Radiographic examination revealed that the second premolar displayed hypercementosis and was located mesially in the position of the missing first premolar. A provisional diagnosis of Paget's disease or fibrous dysplasia was made. Blood was drawn for a full blood count and to test the levels of alkaline phosphatase, calcium, phosphate, growth hormone and glucose, but all were within normal limits. An excisional soft tissue biopsy was attempted, but the lesion recurred within the next month. It again was removed and the underlying bone curetted.

(a) From what three sources is serum alkaline phosphatase derived and how are these distinguished?

(b) Is the patient likely to have Paget's disease or fibrous dysplasia?

(c) Suggest three clinical diagnoses.　·

(d) Comment on the radiograph.

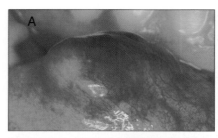

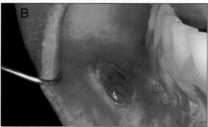

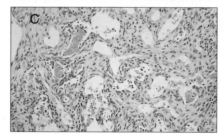

◄ **51** A 19-year-old single hairdresser who was referred by his general dental practitioner because of a painless swelling inside his lower lip. The swelling had been present for about 6 months and was steadily increasing in size.

On examination a large blood-filled swelling was present on the inner aspect of the lip and a provisional diagnosis of a haemangioma was made. Cryotherapy was initiated and resulted in a slight decrease in the size of the lesion but eventually it was decided to excise the lesion. The two photographs are before cryotherapy (A) and 1 month after cryotherapy (B).
(a) What is the principle of cryotherapy?
(b) What clinical effect did cryotherapy have?
(c) Describe the histological appearance of the lesion (C).
(d) Can cryotherapy be detrimental to oral lesions?

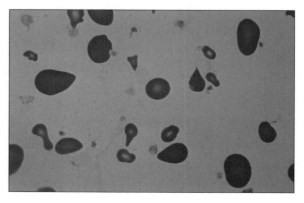

◄ **52** These are red blood cells. With what autoimmune disorder are these changes associated?

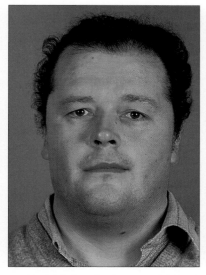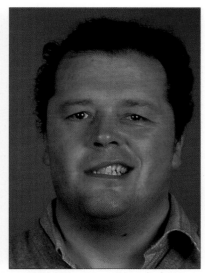

▲ **53** (a) What do these two slides demonstrate?
(b) Is the condition related to diabetes mellitus?
(c) How would you treat the condition?

54 (a) Can the appearance in **53** be caused by varicella zoster?
(b) What is the condition called when caused by varicella zoster?
(c) List six other causes of acute facial nerve palsy.

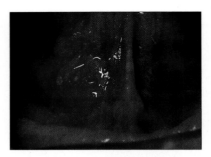

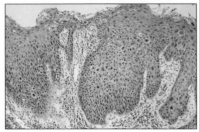

◄ **55** A 53-year-old man was undergoing treatment in a day clinic for alcohol detoxification. He had a 40-year history of smoking 30 cigarettes a day. The patient was hospitalised 5 years ago for hepatitis; he was unsure of the type. Oral examination revealed that the patient was edentulous and at the moment he did not have any dentures. A 30–40 mm lesion was evident on the ventral surface of the tongue. An incisional biopsy was performed. The patient was advised to stop smoking.
(a) What is the likely diagnosis?
(b) What tests should be undertaken prior to biopsy?
(c) Describe the histological features.

▶ **56** A healthy 52-year-old female presented to the Oral Medicine Clinic with a 5-year history of recurrent oral ulceration. The ulcers, located in the anterior part of the mouth, occurred approximately once a month and lasted a few days.

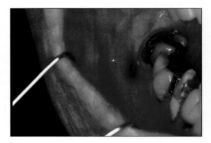

Oral examination revealed asymptomatic geographic tongue and a pigmented lesion on the gingivae in the region of the second molars. The results of routine blood tests, including zinc levels, were normal. The pigmented area was biopsied.
(a) What percentage of (i) Caucasians and (ii) people of colour exhibit intraoral hyperpigmentation?
(b) What is the most important condition to exclude by biopsy?
(c) What is the most likely diagnosis?

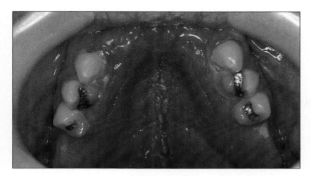

▲ **57** A 27-year-old married development manager was referred by his family doctor because of mouth ulcers he had suffered for several years. He claimed he had never really been clear of ulcers.

There was no relevant medical history. He was partly dentate, with partial upper and lower dentures, and was an irregular dental attender.

The palate had the appearance shown. All blood tests were normal but an oral rinse showed a heavy growth of *Candida albicans.*

(a) What are the two likely diagnoses?

(b) Why do upper partial dentures or other prostheses predispose to erythematous candidiasis?

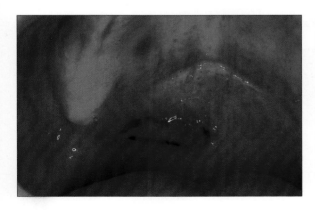

◀ **58** This patient who is otherwise healthy suffers from intermittent sudden onset blood blisters at this site.

(a) What is this condition?

(b) How has it arisen?

(c) Will it recur?

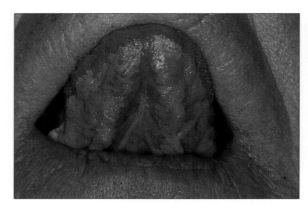

◀ **59** (a) What is this condition? (b) Is it potentially malignant? (c) What management options are available?

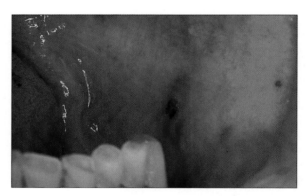

◀ **60** (a) What abnormality is shown? (b) With what blood disorder is this associated?

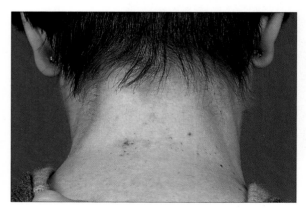

◀ **61** This is the same patient as in **60**. Why have these lesions developed at this site?

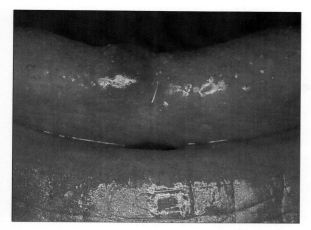

▲ **62** The patient, a 70-year-old retired housewife, was on thyroxine therapy only. She presented with a painless lesion on the tip of her tongue which had been there for about 2 years. The lesion was excised and submitted for microscopic study.

(a) What is the significance of the colour of the lesion?
(b) Would any preoperative investigations be helpful?
(c) Would steroid cover be required at the time of operation?

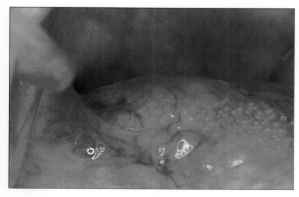

▲ **63** (a) What is this structure?
(b) Is it potentially malignant?
(c) Is any treatment necessary?

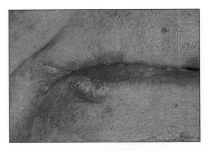

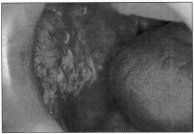

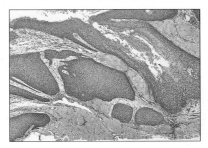

◄ **64** A 69-year-old man was referred because of a slowly expanding, painless lesion of 1 year's duration on the right side of the lower lip.

The patient had a gastric ulcer that perforated several months ago, for which he was prescribed cimetidine. He also took albuterol 4 mg four times a day for his bronchitis. The patient was retired and married; he had smoked 20 cigarettes a day for the past 60 years and drank four whiskies a day. He had been edentulous for 50 years and his present dentures were 8 or 9 years old.

On oral examination an indurated mass was detected on the lower lip near the right commissure. Intraorally, the right buccal mucosa was covered by a leukoplakic patch that extended onto the soft palate. Incisional biopsies were performed on the lip and right buccal mucosa.
(a) What is the likely clinical diagnosis of the lip lesion?
(b) Discuss the salient histological features of the lip lesion.
(c) What is the treatment of choice?
(d) What is the long-term prognosis?

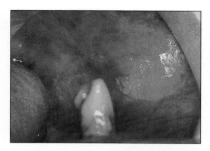

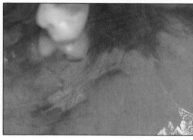

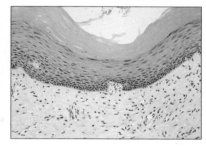

◀ **65** This 59-year-old retired man self-referred to Casualty with toothache, which resulted in extractions. Asymptomatic white patches were noted on the right and left buccal mucosa, palate and alveolar ridge.

Medically he suffered from angina and used glyceryl trinitrate sublingual sprays. Previous operations include a prostate operation and a hernia repair. He had smoked 25–30 cigarettes a day for the past 35 years and claimed a moderate alcohol intake.

Clinical examination revealed an edentulous upper ridge and partially dentate lower, with reticular white patches on the buccal mucosa, palate and edentulous alveolar ridge. An incisional biopsy on the left buccal mucosa was performed.

(a) Irregular dental attenders pose a particular problem in the management of mucosal lesions – why?

(b) Are the adverse oral effects of smoking and alcohol additive?

(c) Is dental disease a risk factor in oral cancer?

(d) From the histological appearance of the lesion what is the diagnosis?

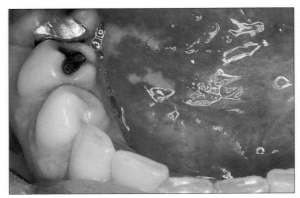

◄ **66** These lesions are 2 days old.
(a) What kind of aphthous ulceration is this?
(b) Is it commoner in women or in men?

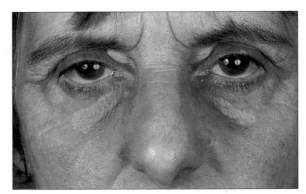

◄ **67** (a) What is this condition?
(b) What is its cause?
(c) What blood tests are indicated?

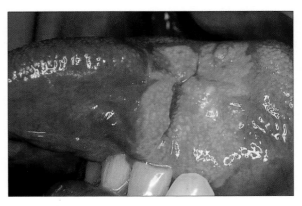

◄ **68** (a) From what condition has this patient suffered?
(b) How do you know the white area is the result of treatment?
(c) What clinical features suggest infection?

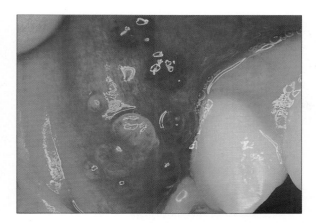

▲ **69** A healthy 14-year-old boy's chief complaint was of asymptomatic multilobular elevated areas on the right maxillary labial mucosa. A mucosal biopsy was performed.
(a) What is the likely clinical diagnosis?
(b) What treatment options are available?
(c) In which part of the body are these lesions most likely to be seen?
(d) What age group is most frequently affected?

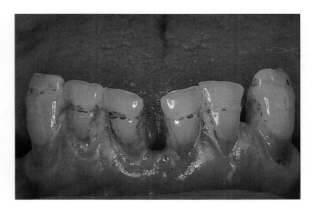

◀ **70** (a) What has caused these lesions on the crowns of the lower incisors and canines?
(b) Around what age did this event occur?

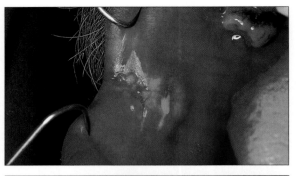

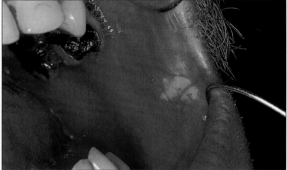

▲ 71 A 41-year-old security officer referred by his doctor had a 4-month history of a rough lump on the inside of his right cheek. The area was painful whenever he was eating hard food.

The patient was hypertensive, for which he took propranolol and amiloride. He also took lorazepam once a day for his nerves and had been treated in the past for depression. He was married, smoked 40 cigarettes a day, and currently was a non-drinker but had a history of previous alcohol abuse.

Oral examination revealed inadequate oral hygiene and erythema of the palatal region covered by a partial denture. On the buccal mucosa, just behind the right and left commissures, white areas approximately 5 mm in diameter were observed. The right one was somewhat elevated and ulcerated, and was biopsied. At the first visit routine haematological and microbiological investigations were conducted.

(a) What is the likely diagnosis?
(b) Give three predisposing factors.
(c) What management regime is likely to be effective?

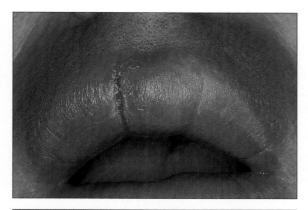

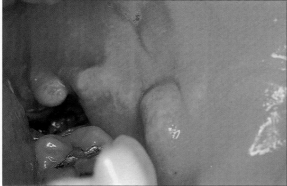

▲ **72** A 32-year-old medically fit married man presented because of a swollen upper lip, of 1 year's duration, that occasionally cracked. Intraorally the buccal mucosa appeared oedematous with large mucosal elevations that were hyperkeratotic, possibly because of trauma from adjacent teeth.

The patient smoked about 50 cigarettes a day, drank 10 pints of beer on the weekends and had three to four bottles of a soft drink and two to three curries per week.

Routine blood tests were normal, but a radioallergosorbent test (RAST) was positive for grass pollen. A biopsy of the buccal mucosa down to the buccinator muscle was subsequently performed.

(a) What is the likely diagnosis?
(b) What is the significance of the patient's dietary habits on the disorder?
(c) Is the positive RAST test significant?
(d) What is the prognosis?

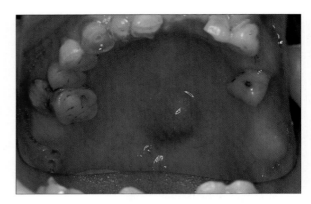

◄ **73** (a) Is this likely to be a benign or malignant salivary gland tumour?
(b) If malignant, what kind of histology is most likely?
(c) What is the prognosis?

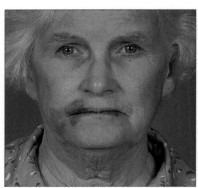

◄ **74** This lady has no history of trauma.
(a) What abnormality is shown?
(b) List four possible serious underlying conditions.

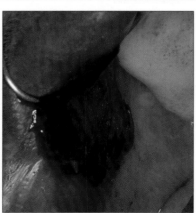

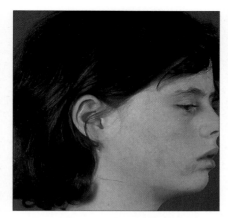

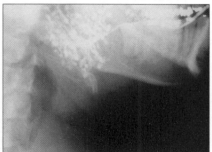

75 (a) What do these two slides demonstrate?
(b) What is the diagnosis?
(c) How should it be managed?

76 (a) What is this condition?
(b) Is it potentially malignant?
(c) Name three predisposing factors.

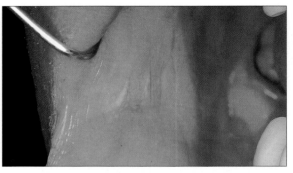

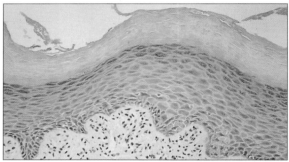

▲ 77 A 43-year-old man presented with a 10-year complaint of cracking in the corners of his mouth. The condition was intermittent; it would undergo periods of spontaneous remission but then recur.

His medical history revealed treatment for sinusitis. The patient smoked one ounce (28 g) of tobacco per week in the form of roll-ups.

A diagnosis of angular cheilitis was made and investigations included routine blood and microbiological tests. Investigations also revealed slight iron deficiency, for which he subsequently received adequate iron replacement therapy. A light candidal growth was treated with a variety of topical agents. Systemic antifungal therapy with fluconazole finally eliminated the problem.

At his review, 6 months later, a painful lesion inside the angle of his mouth was discovered and biopsied.

(a) Give three differential diagnoses for a lesion at this site.
(b) What could be the relationship between the original condition of angular cheilitis and the present lesion?
(c) Are angular cheilitis and iron deficiency related?
(d) What are the main histological features present?
(e) Based on the histopathologic findings what is the prognosis?

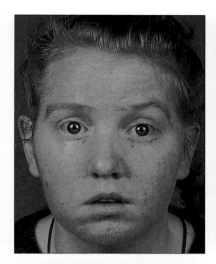
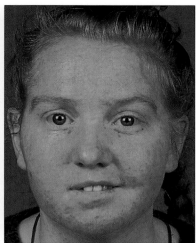
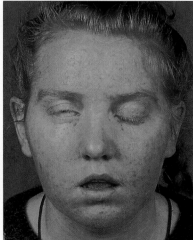

▲ ◀ **78** This healthy 15-year-old girl developed an inability to move the muscles on one side of her face. The condition developed over a period of several hours and was not preceded by trauma. She presented the same day to the Oral Medicine Clinic.

(a) What is the likely diagnosis?

(b) How would you treat the condition?

(c) These photographs were taken 2 weeks after initial presentation. What skin condition has developed and why?

(d) What is the prognosis for the facial muscle problem?

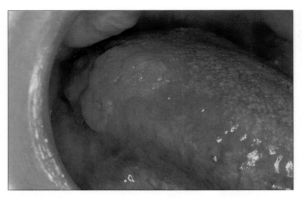

▲ 79 This is a squamous cell carcinoma.
(a) Is the prognosis better or worse if the patient does not smoke and does not drink alcohol?
(b) Name the main staging system used to assess these lesions?
(c) Overall, what is the 5-year survival from oral cancer?

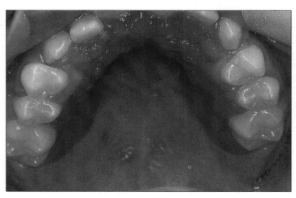

▲ 80 (a) What is this condition?
(b) Why has it developed in this dentate patient?

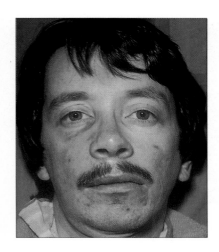

81 This man has glandular fever. What has caused the appearance below his right eye?

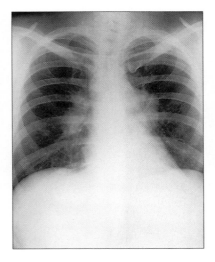

82 This 39-year-old male presented with bilateral sublingual gland swelling of 2 months' duration. He had no medical history of note apart from alopecia areata and did not smoke or drink. He also complained of eye discomfort and breathlessness. A right buccal mucosal biopsy and this chest radiograph were taken.

(a) What key histological feature would you expect?
(b) What is the likely diagnosis?
(c) What is demonstrated on the chest radiograph?
(d) What other investigations may be helpful?
(e) What is the prognosis?

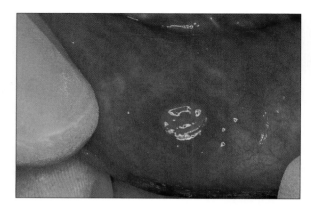

83 (a) What is this condition? (b) With what deficiency states is it associated? (c) How would you manage it?

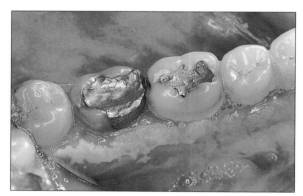

84 (a) Is this a lichenoid reaction? (b) Would biopsy be helpful? (c) Are the adjacent amalgam fillings relevant?

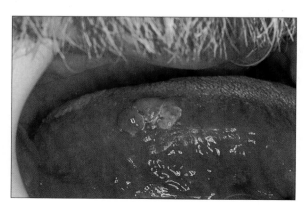

85 What three factors would concern you about this lesion?

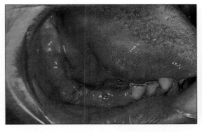
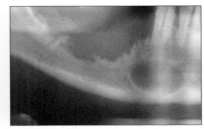
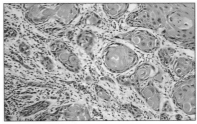

▲ **86** This 38-year-old single mother of a 4-month-old baby presented complaining of chronic pain with bleeding in the lower right jaw, the extraction site of five teeth removed 5 weeks earlier. She also complained of swelling in the right submandibular and submental regions and apparently had lost 4 kg in weight since the extractions. She was taking paracetamol (acetaminophen) for the discomfort. She smoked heavily, perhaps 40 cigarettes a day, and admitted to drinking alcohol on a social basis. At the time of her examination the aroma of alcohol on her breath was very strong.

Clinical and radiographic examinations were performed. The patient was partially dentate with poor oral hygiene. An erythematous fleshy growth was noted in the mandibular right canine to molar region and an incisional biopsy was performed.
(a) What two main radiological features are evident?
(b) What is the histological diagnosis?
(c) What management options are available?

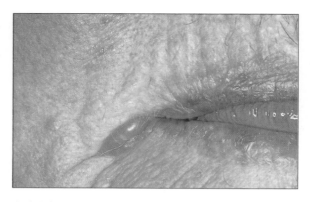

▲ **87** A 71-year-old single woman, a retired secretary, was referred by her medical practitioner because of a non-painful area at the right commissure of the lip. The lesion had persisted for approximately 2 years in spite of topical application of antibiotic creams.

The patient for many years suffered from 'rheumatism' in her shoulders and took diazepam to aid sleep. In her youth she had been a heavy smoker but had stopped 30 years ago. She drank alcohol on occasion. Fully edentulous for 50 years, her current dentures were 1 year old.

On examination bilateral angular cheilitis and an elevated lesion at the right commissural region were noted. Routine haematological investigations were within the normal range and microbiological investigations revealed a moderate growth of *Candida albicans* from an oral rinse. An incisional biopsy from the region of the right commissure was made.

(a) Is it appropriate to treat an edentulous patient for 'angular cheilitis' with antibiotic creams?

(b) If the patient had angular cheilitis and candidal species were isolated from the oral cavity what test would prove that these were the same species of organism?

(c) What is the differential diagnosis?

(d) How may the medical condition have contributed to the condition?

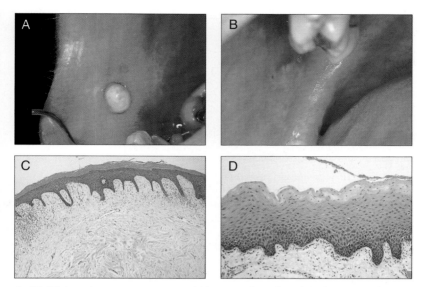

▲ **88** This patient was a 42-year-old housewife, referred by her general dental practitioner, complaining of a growth in the right buccal mucosa and white areas on the buccal mucosa.

Medical history revealed she suffered from psoriasis and was taking treatment for this. She smoked 10 cigarettes per day and drank half a bottle of vodka a week. She was dentate and an irregular attender.

An excision biopsy was undertaken of the polyp in the right buccal mucosa and an incisional biopsy was taken of the right buccal mucosa adjacent to the molar teeth.

(a) Does psoriasis affect the oral mucosa?

(b) Why is the polypoid lesion so white in appearance?

(c) Comment on the histological features of the polypoid lesion (**C**) and suggest a diagnosis.

(d) Comment on the histological features of the buccal lesion (**D**) and suggest a diagnosis.

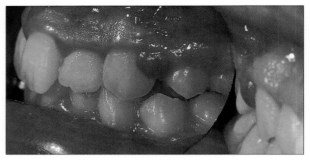

▲ **89** This 12-year-old girl presented with the complaint of 'the gum growing down between two of her upper left teeth'. The growth was first noted some months before. It now was fairly stable in size but bled on occasion. The medical history was non-contributory.

On examination the interdental papilla between the upper left canine and first premolar was soft, cyanotic and enlarged. The lesion was removed by surgical excision.

(a) Is this lesion likely to be a haemangioma?

(b) Would preoperative radiographs have been helpful?

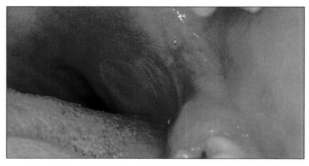

▲ **90** A 10-year-old girl had suffered from recurrent mouth ulcers for about 10 years. The ulcers were usually at the posterior aspect of her mouth in the soft palate/faucial region and (untreated) took 4–6 weeks to heal. She was otherwise in good health.

(a) How are aphthous ulcers classified?

(b) What haematinic deficiency states are known to be associated with aphthous ulceration?

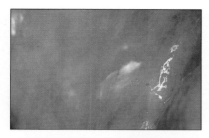

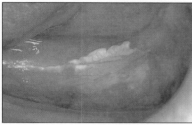

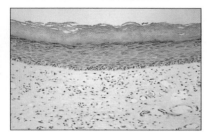

◀ **91** A 71-year-old widowed housewife was referred by her dentist because of intraoral white lesions of unknown duration. The patient did not smoke or drink alcohol. She had had rheumatic fever at the age of 13 years. Edentulous, she had difficulty wearing complete dentures.

On oral examination a white patch was observed on the right buccal mucosa just inferior to the parotid orifice; a second extensive white area covered much of the right mandibular alveolar ridge. Microbiological and routine haematological investigations revealed no abnormalities. A biopsy of the right buccal mucosa was undertaken.

(a) Why was the buccal mucosa biopsied instead of the alveolar ridge?

(b) Would the patient be biopsied under antibiotic cover?

(c) What are the salient histological features?

92 Define and list six causes of sialosis.

93 (a) Is hairy leukoplakia of prognostic significance?
(b) Is the condition pathognomonic of HIV infection?

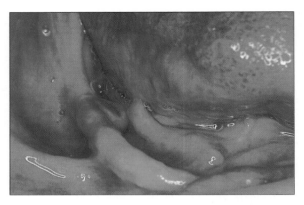

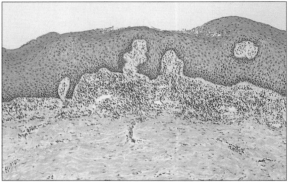

▲ 94 A 47-year-old married auxiliary nurse was referred by her general dental practitioner regarding a hyperplastic nodule in the right lower alveolar region lingually. A similar lesion had been removed by another dental surgeon in the practice several months previously but the condition recurred.

Medical history revealed current medication to be hormone replacement therapy only. She wore complete upper and lower dentures that were 10 years old and worn continuously. An excisional biopsy was performed.

(a) What is the likely clinical diagnosis?

(b) Comment on the histological features.

(c) What steps could be taken to prevent another recurrence?

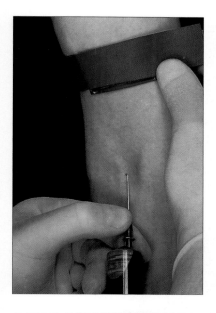

◀ **95** (a) What is the main danger to the doctor from venepuncture?
(b) What is this region of the arm called?
(c) Do haemophiliacs bleed excessively following venepuncture?

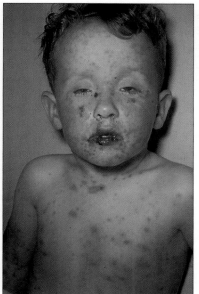

◀ **96** This child has primary herpetic gingivostomatitis.
(a) What medical condition may have made his condition worse?
(b) What drug therapy would you advise?

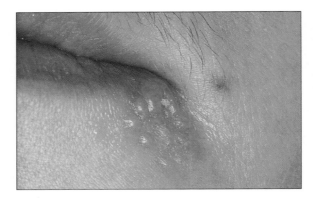

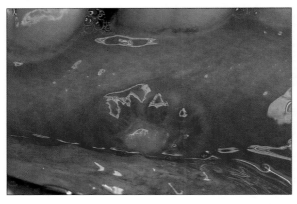

▲ 98 A 40-year-old married radiographer who was a regular dental attender was referred by his general dental practitioner regarding a chronic 'ulcer' of 1 month's duration on the lingual gingiva/alveolar mucosa of the mandibular right first molar (mirror view).

Medically he was taking chlordiazepoxide and had a penicillin allergy but was otherwise well. Oral examination revealed a discharging sinus to the lingual of the first molar.

Radiographic examination revealed a radiolucent area around the distal root of the same tooth. A full-thickness flap was reflected and a piece of the lingual cortical plate of bone removed and sent for microscopic examination. A 5-day course of metronidazole was prescribed and the patient's dentist was asked to undertake root canal therapy or extraction of the first molar.

(a) What is the likely diagnosis?
(b) Is the patient's occupation relevant?

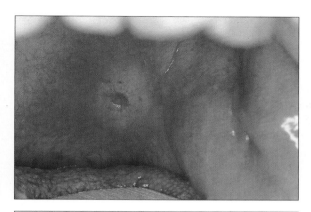

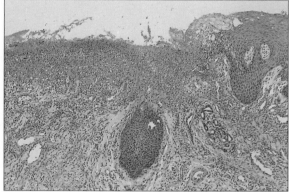

▲ **99** This 63-year-old woman presented to the Oral Medicine Department complaining of a small ulcer on the palate, which had been present for 6 weeks. The patient was a non-insulin dependent diabetic under good control. She suffered from depression, primarily due to the recent death of her husband, for which she took 5 mg of diazepam and 75 mg of a tricyclic antidepressant daily.

Oral examination revealed a small ulcer on the soft palate. A provisional diagnosis of a traumatic ulcer was made. Routine microbiological and haematological tests were normal. No treatment was given but when the patient returned 2 weeks later and the ulcer had not resolved, an excisional biopsy was performed.
(a) Describe the histological features seen.
(b) Can you speculate on the role of diabetes mellitus in the development of the lesion?
(c) Could the lesion be self-inflicted?

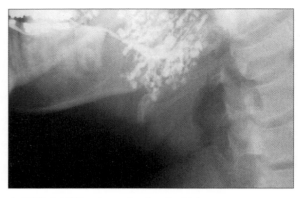

▲ **100** (a) What investigation is this?
(b) What two diagnoses are most likely?
(c) What gives rise to the appearance seen?

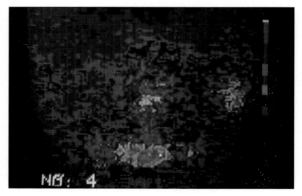

▲ **101** A 28-year-old vet had self-prescribed
antibiotics for 4 years for recurrent parotid gland
infections. She was in good health and was finally
persuaded to seek a dental opinion.
(a) What investigation is this?
(b) What does it show?
(c) Suggest two treatment options.

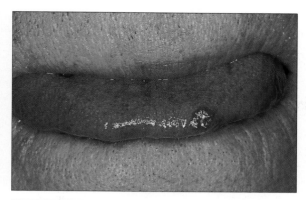

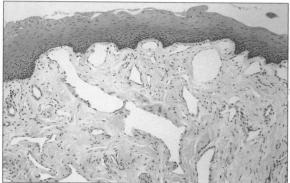

▲ 102 A 76-year-old male married retired maintenance worker was referred by his general dental practitioner regarding lumps on his tongue that he described as blisters and which had been there for 6 months.

Medically he had angina for which he took glyceryl trinitrate. A biopsy of the left tip of the dorsum of the tongue was undertaken.

(a) Would a full blood count be helpful?

(b) Describe the histological features. What is the diagnosis?

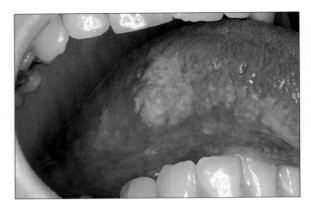

103 (a) What is this condition?
(b) What is the most important clinical feature evident?
(c) What do the anterior lesions signify?

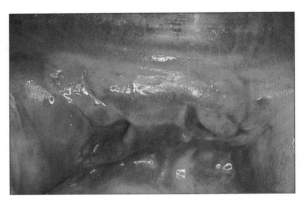

104 These lesions are on the inner aspect of the lower lip. What do you think caused these lesions and why?

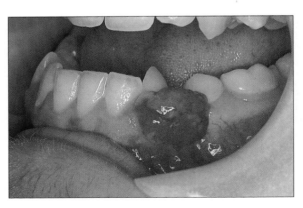

105 This patient is not pregnant.
(a) List three differential diagnoses.
(b) What blood tests are appropriate?
(c) What radiographs are appropriate?

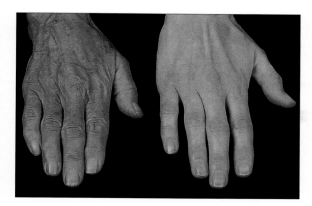

◀ 106 Both patients are Caucasians. Name two pathological conditions associated with generalised pigmentation.

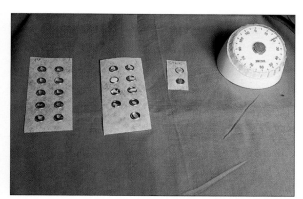

◀ 107 (a) What is this investigation? (b) List six orofacial diseases in which it has value.

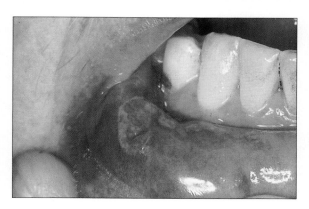

◀ 108 This patient claimed to have bitten her lip.
(a) What clinical sign suggests serious underlying disease?
(b) What blood tests are appropriate?
(c) What treatment would you advise?

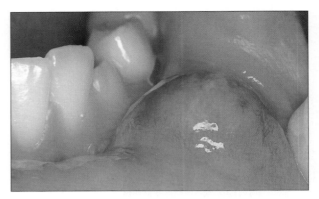

▲ **109** A 12-year-old schoolgirl with no relevant medical history had a 3-month history of an increasing and a decreasing swelling in the lower lip, apparently associated with trauma. The large soft cyanotic swelling was excised under local anaesthesia.
(a) What is the likely diagnosis?
(b) What is the usual histological appearance?
(c) Is there a relationship between this lesion and trauma?

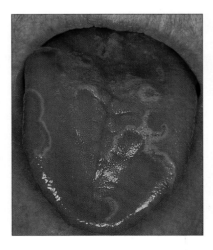

◀ **110** (a) What is this condition?
(b) Is it inherited?
(c) What causes the condition?

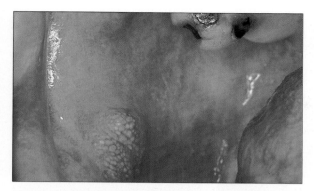

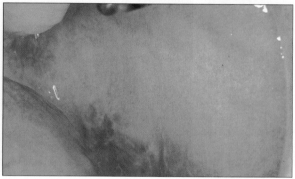

▲ 111 This 64-year-old health worker drank socially but did not smoke; her chief complaint was a painful region on the right buccal mucosa for the past 8 weeks. The patient suffered from bronchiectasis and rheumatoid arthritis. She was taking an antiarrhythmic drug and was allergic to ampicillin. Four years ago she had a hip replacement.

The oral examination revealed subtle white striae and atrophic areas on both the right and left buccal mucosa. A rough speckled swelling (approximately 6 mm in diameter) found on the right buccal mucosa was removed.
(a) What condition would be most likely in this patient given the bilateral distribution of her lesions?
(b) What diagnosis does the appearance of the right buccal mucosa suggest?
(c) How should the patient be managed?

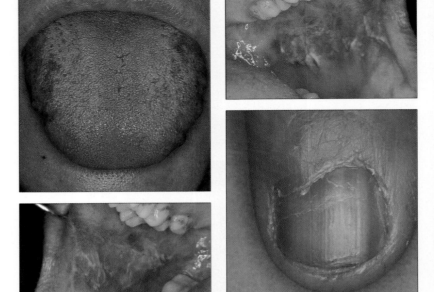

▲ **112** The patient, a 42-year-old housewife, presented complaining of burning of her mouth and tongue on eating hot and spicy foods. She suffered from rheumatoid arthritis and asthma. Clinical features are as shown, with pigmented areas on both buccal mucosae and both lateral margins of the tongue. Her nails were also pigmented. The buccal mucosal lesions were of reticular lichen planus.

(a) What name is given to this pigmented condition?
(b) Is it inherited?
(c) What is the prognosis?

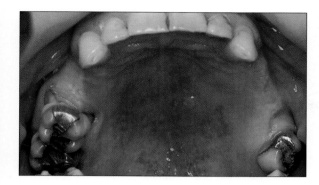

◄ **113** (a) What kind of oral candidiasis is this?
(b) List six predisposing factors.
(c) The patient is diabetic – is this relevant?

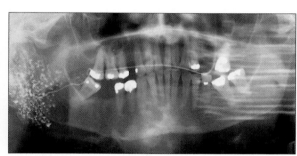

◄ **114** (a) What investigation is being undertaken?
(b) What is the disadvantage of this technique?

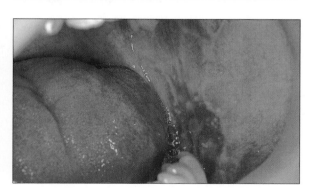

◄ **115** How would you determine if this was erosive lichen planus or discoid lupus erythematosus?

116 (a) Does it matter if the diagnosis of **115** is lichen planus or discoid lupus erythematosus?
(b) Are antinuclear factor levels useful in diagnosis?

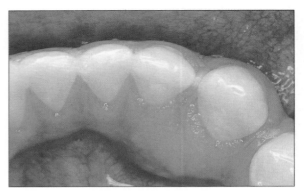

▲ **117** This healthy 15-year-old boy was referred because of a swelling behind the lower front teeth which had been present for about 1 year. It was non-painful and there was little recent change in size. The patient smoked 10–20 cigarettes a day and drank alcohol on occasion. On examination there was a hard swelling lingual to the lower left lateral and canine teeth that was slightly painful to palpation. A mucoperiosteal flap was raised and a small bony protrusion was seen. The superficial layer of bone was removed, revealing a small sinus which was curetted. This material was sent for microscopic examination.
(a) What clinical evidence is there that the lesion is not infective?
(b) Can periapical pathology be found in teeth with clinically normal crowns?

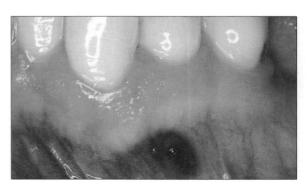

◀ **118** (a) What is this condition?
(b) Would a radiograph be helpful?
(c) What is the main differential diagnosis?

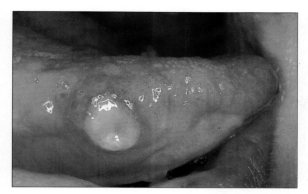

▲ **119** A woman in her 30s suffered from cyclic neutropenia, recurrent oral ulceration, iron deficiency anaemia and possible inflammatory bowel disease. She did not smoke but drank alcohol occasionally. She had been receiving systemic steroids for a decade but when weaned off the medication there was an exacerbation of her oral ulceration.

(a) How would you confirm the diagnosis of cyclic neutropenia?

(b) What other oral problems do patients with cyclic neutropenia have?

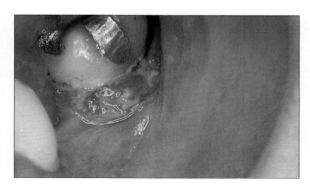

◀ **120** (a) If this is a pyogenic granuloma, what may have precipitated it?

(b) What is your main differential diagnosis?

(c) Would a radiograph be helpful?

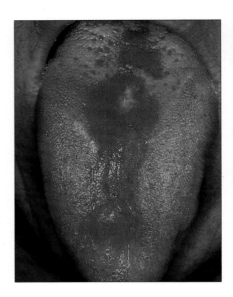

◄ **121** (a) What is this condition?
(b) What is it caused by?
(c) What drug has precipitated it?

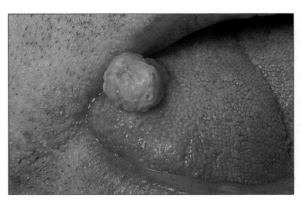

◄ **122** This is a
benign neoplasm.
List the potential
tissues of origin.

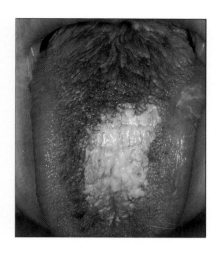

◀ **123** This patient has tertiary syphilis.
(a) What is this lesion called?
(b) From what other tongue condition does the patient suffer?

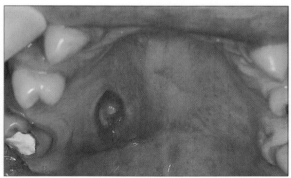

◀ **124** This ulcer was preceded by paraesthesia.
(a) What is the condition called?
(b) How is it related to the dressed tooth?

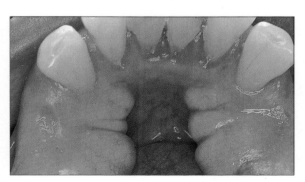

◀ **125** (a) What are these called?
(b) Name two conditions with which they are associated.

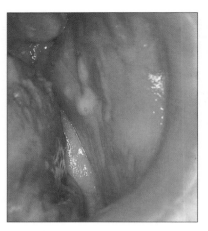

◀ **126** This patient was 40 years old and in good health. Over the previous 3 years she had been prescribed systemic antibiotics on five occasions for a painful preauricular swelling.

(a) What does this clinical photograph demonstrate?

(b) What is this condition called?

(c) What organisms are involved?

(d) If the condition resolved with further antibiotic therapy what investigation is then warranted?

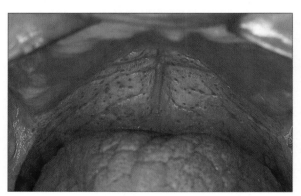

◀ **127** (a) What is this condition?

(b) Is it potentially malignant?

(c) What causes the condition?

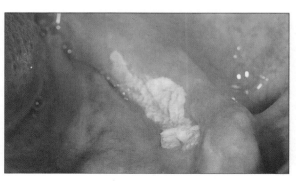

◀ **128** (a) How would you biopsy this lesion?

(b) Would you use resorbable or non-resorbable sutures?

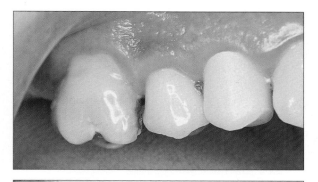

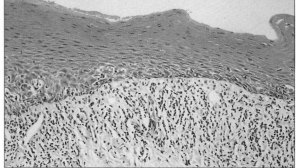

▲ **129** This 55-year-old married shop assistant was a non-smoker, originally referred by her family dentist for management of temporomandibular joint pain. On examination a lesion was noted in the upper right quadrant, which was thought to have been present for about 6 months.

Her medical history revealed that she was fit and well apart from receiving therapy for high blood pressure. Her dental history showed she was a regular attender. On examination there was an erythematous and tender area on the upper right quadrant, which appeared traumatic at the time. This was subsequently biopsied.

(a) Describe the main clinical features.

(b) What is the clinical diagnosis?

(c) Would any blood tests be helpful?

(d) Discuss the histological features evident.

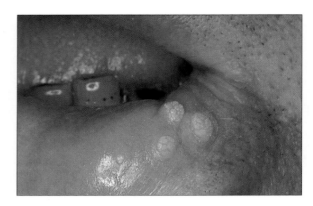

◀ **130** (a) What are these lesions? (b) What is their cause? (c) What is the likely source of infection?

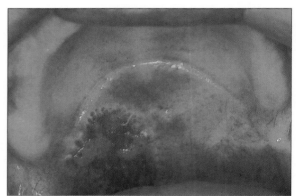

◀ **131** (a) Why is this not erythroplakia? (b) What investigations would you undertake?

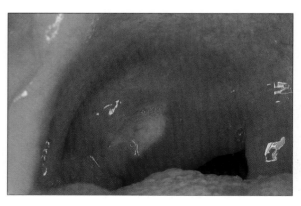

◀ **132** (a) Is this the most common site for major aphthae? (b) How would you determine if the patient had Behçet's disease?

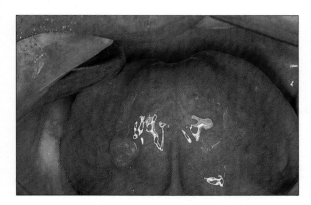

◀ **133** (a) What is this condition? (b) His brother had the same condition – is that significant?

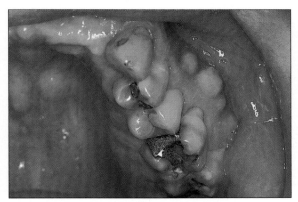

◀ **134** (a) What are these lesion? (b) Do they appear on radiographs? (c) Are they associated with any syndrome?

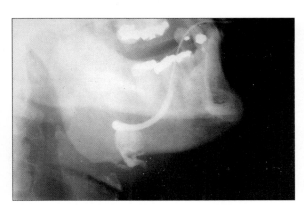

◀ **135** (a) What investigation is this? (b) What gland is being investigated? (c) What abnormality is shown?

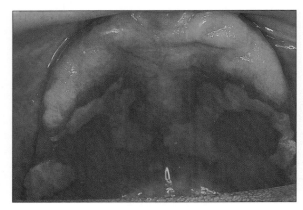

136 (a) Name the group of mucosal disorders that most affect the hard and soft palate.
(b) What are your two main differential diagnoses?
(c) What single laboratory investigation is most helpful in these cases?

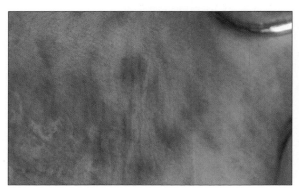

137 (a) What is the commonest cause of oral pigmentation?
(b) How would you exclude Addison's disease?

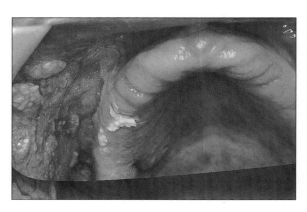

138 (a) What is this condition?
(b) If surgically excised, could similar lesions develop in other sites in the mouth?

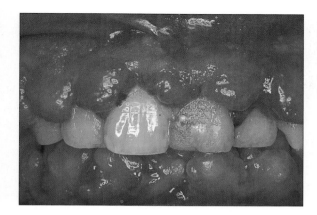

◀ **139** (a) List six causes of this condition.
(b) Why is it more severe in the lower arch?

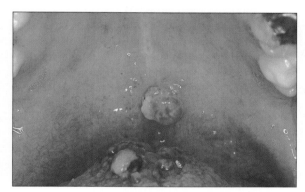

◀ **140** These lesions have the same microscopic appearance.
(a) What is the causative process?
(b) Is biopsy advisable?

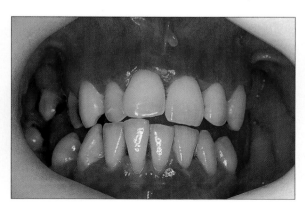

◀ **141** (a) What is this condition?
(b) Name two diseases with which it is associated.
(c) How would you treat it?

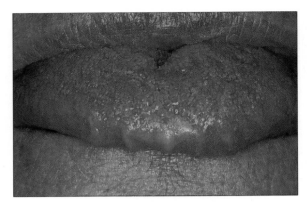

◄ **142** (a) What abnormality is shown?
(b) What has caused this condition?
(c) What symptoms might the patient have?

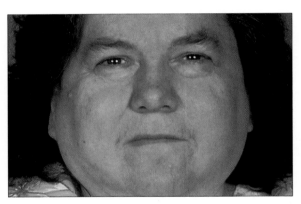

◄ **143** What salivary abnormality is demonstrated?

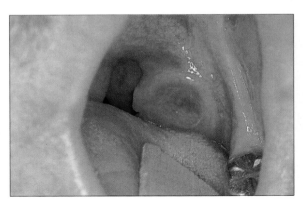

◄ **144** (a) What kind of tumour is this?
(b) Is it associated with underlying disease?
(c) What is the prognosis?

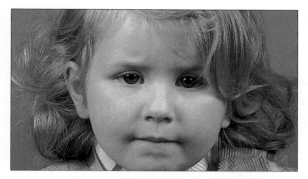

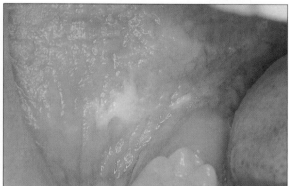

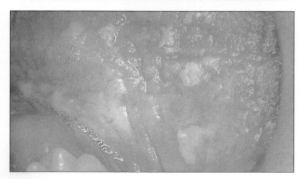

▲ **145** This young girl had these lesions in her mouth.
(a) What is the diagnosis?
(b) What drugs can be used to treat the condition?

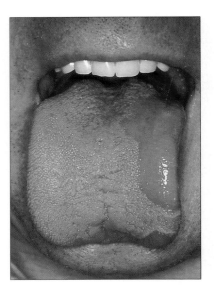

◄ **146** (a) What is this condition? (b) What skin condition do the histological features resemble?

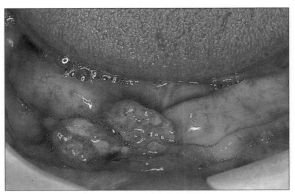

◄ **147** (a) Why is this not a denture-induced hyperplasia? (b) What is the likely diagnosis?

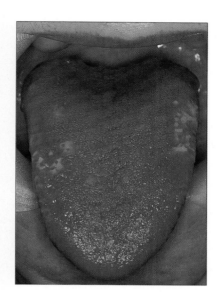

◀ **148** (a) What is this condition? (b) What would your management be?

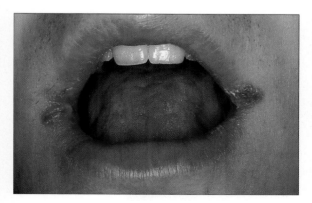

◀ **149** (a) What is this condition called? (b) What organisms are usually responsible? (c) What would your management be?

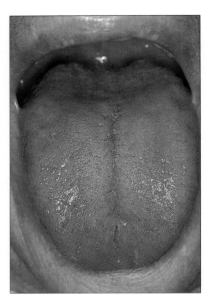

◀ **150** This patient complained of a constant burning sensation of the tongue. List twelve causes of a persistent burning sensation in a healthy looking tongue.

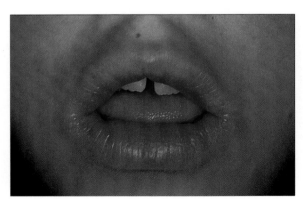

◀ **151** (a) What is this condition?
(b) How is it related to bowel disease?
(c) What is it caused by?

ANSWERS

1   (a) Squamous cell papilloma.
(b) Localised, well-circumscribed lesion, very white in appearance with a cauliflower-like appearance. These are all typical features of a squamous cell papilloma.
(c) Heck's disease.
(d) Human papilloma virus can frequently be demonstrated by in-situ hybridisation. The types involved are usually types 6, 11, 13, 16 and 32.
(e) No. These lesions are entirely benign.

2   (a) Grinspan's syndrome is the name given to the triad of diabetes mellitus, essential hypertension and oral lichen planus. It would appear that in most cases of Grinspan's syndrome the oral lesions are lichenoid secondary to drug therapy rather than idiopathic lichen planus.
(b) Antihypertensive drugs and analgesics (in this case unspecified) can both give rise to oral lichenoid reactions. Usually lichenoid reactions are unilateral, but they can be bilateral and mimic lichen planus, perhaps as in this case.
(c) The epithelium covering the swelling looks clinically normal and, therefore, the pathological process is submucosal. Likely candidates in this process include neoplasms of neural tissue, muscle and adipose tissue but occasionally localised deposits of amyloid can be clinically indistinguishable. This was a neurolemmoma.

3   (a) Gingival fibrous overgrowth, hamartoma, neural tumour.
(b) Possibly. This patient was on no steroid treatment for asthma but did use hydrocortisone cream for her eczema. The extent of her eczema and dose of hydrocortisone used would dictate the need for steroid cover. Clearly, if large areas of her skin had eczema and she used copious amounts of hydrocortisone then steroid cover would be advisable.

4   (a) Dyskeratosis congenita, pachyonychia congenita, white sponge naevus, mucocutaneous candidiasis.
(b) White sponge naevus. The other conditions are much rarer and, in the absence of nail lesions, systemic upset or immunological abnormality are effectively excluded.
(c) Autosomal dominant with incomplete penetrance and variable expressivity.
(d) Rarely involvement of the nasal, rectal or genital mucosa occurs in cases of white sponge naevus.

5   (a) No. Psychological disorders have never been proven to produce persistent xerostomia. The dorsum of the tongue is obviously very dry and there is also mucosal atrophy, probably indicating the long-standing nature of the complaint.
(b) No. Diazepam or other benzodiazepines have no proven effect on salivary gland function. Indeed in the elderly the opposite is the case, with excessive salivation – a response also occasionally noted in children.
(c) No. Chronic alcohol abuse can affect the major salivary glands but the outcome is sialosis. Sialosis is a non-inflammatory, non-neoplastic enlargement of (usually) the parotid glands. Chronic alcoholism is known to produce sialosis but although the glands are clinically enlarged their function is not reduced. However, the

dorsum of this patient's tongue is atrophic. With this degree of mucosal atrophy two aetiological factors are likely, either xerostomia or nutritional deficiency. In this case no haematinic deficiency state was detected and the mucosal atrophy is presumably only due to xerostomia.

(d) Yes. Patients with clinically obvious long-standing xerostomia almost invariably have intraoral candidal carriage and/or infection. An oral rinse is the only way to quantify this carriage. Most of the oral discomfort in patients with xerostomia is due to *Candida* and eradication by antifungal therapy can produce considerable symptomatic relief, even though salivary flow is unchanged.

(e) A labial gland biopsy to confirm or exclude Sjögren's syndrome. In a known alcoholic the production of blood coagulation factors by the liver is likely to be impaired and a coagulation screen should be undertaken prior to biopsy. Advice from a consultant haematologist should be sought to correct any abnormality detected. One clinical precaution that should be taken is to ensure the labial gland biopsy is adequate (i.e. at least five lobules taken from below an area of clinically normal mucosa). Mucosal pathosis can produce histological changes in minor salivary glands, which make interpretation difficult.

(f) Rheumatoid factor is an antibody against the patient's own immunoglobulin. It is commonly positive in rheumatoid arthritis (the patient being termed sero-positive) and can be positive in systemic lupus erythematosus, systemic sclerosis and primary biliary cirrhosis.

6   (a) Squamous cell carcinoma. An elevated lesion on the posterior aspect of the tongue in an elderly patient who smokes must be regarded as highly suspicious.

(b) The first biopsy shows non-specific chronic ulceration. There is a break in the continuity of the epithelium and the surface comprises fibrin and enmeshed inflammatory cells. The epithelium at the margin of the ulcer shows some reactive changes, but there is no dysplasia.

(c) Occasionally, in patients who have obvious oral squamous cell carcinoma, the initial biopsy fails to detect oral malignancy. Presumably in these cases the wrong area has been biopsied. In this case, the lesion 1 week later showed no signs of healing and looked clinically even more sinister than at first. Therefore, a repeat excisional biopsy was performed.

(d) The features are similar to the first biopsy and show non-specific chronic ulceration. The base of the ulcer is granulation tissue, but the healing response does not appear particularly vigorous.

(e) Cases of non-specific chronic ulceration that look clinically very serious are puzzling. They usually occur in elderly patients. There could be underlying ischaemia precipitating the lesions and giving the poor healing but, in truth, the cause is unknown. It would be wise to review the patient every 6 months to check for recurrence or new lesion formation.

7   (a) No. Iron deficiency is not a disease but a manifestation of inadequate dietary intake, malabsorption or excess loss or utilisation. Occult neoplasia in the gastrointestinal or renal/urinary tract can lead to iron deficiency even in the absence

of symptoms. In a patient of this age group a dietary history, questioning as to blood (fresh or otherwise) in faeces, and urinalysis would all be required. The fact that routine haematological investigations, such as a full blood picture, were normal effectively excludes increased iron utilisation due to haematological malignancy, such as leukaemia. If all investigations are normal then, in a patient of this age group, dietary deficiency of iron is likely and oral iron therapy should be given. Iron therapy needs to be prolonged (i.e. several months) and repeat measurement of ferritin would be necessary to ensure levels have returned to normal.

(b) Sideropenia (i.e. reduced iron levels in the absence of anaemia) produces epithelial atrophy. There are reports of patients with lesions such as seen in this case resolving entirely with iron-replacement therapy. Others have reported a similar phenomenon in patients with vitamin B_{12} deficiency.

(c) The epithelium is atrophic and heavily keratinised. Mild epithelial dysplasia is present, confined to the deeper layers of the epithelium. Non-specific chronic inflammatory cell infiltration is present in the lamina propria.

(d) Encouraging cessation of smoking and moderation in alcohol intake should be the first steps in management. Iron-replacement therapy alone may resolve the clinical damage. Repeat biopsy at 3 months is recommended.

8   (a) Two known ocular complications of mucous membrane pemphigoid are symblepharon and glaucoma. Symblepharon is characterised by surface corneal scarring, which can produce blindness. Glaucoma is painless raised intraocular pressure, which can also lead to loss of vision.

(b) The respiratory infection one would be most concerned about being reactivated by high-dose, long-term corticosteroid therapy is tuberculosis. For this reason, patients who are on long-term, high-dose steroid therapy have annual chest X-rays to evaluate any possible recurrence of tuberculosis.

(c) Pemphigus vulgaris was previously fatal before the onset of steroid therapy because of widespread skin loss leading to fluid imbalance and also bacterial infection and septicaemia. With the advent of corticosteroid therapy, pemphigus is no longer considered a fatal disease.

9   Three benefits of acyclovir cream are:

(a) prevention of the lesion progressing beyond the prodromal stage in about 50% of patients;

(b) a marked reduction in the size of the lesion in patients who do develop the condition. Indeed, about 44% of patients have a lesion reduced in size by about 80% ;

(c) of the patients who do develop lesions of normal size, healing time is decreased by approximately 1.5 days.

10   (a) Actinic keratosis and squamous cell carcinoma. The elevated nature of the lesion would favour the diagnosis of carcinoma, perhaps arising out of an area of actinic keratosis.

(b) There is prominent hyperkeratosis. The epithelium shows moderate dysplasia, but there is no evidence of invasion. The underlying connective tissue has a rather uniform eosinophilic appearance and this area would stain positively with elastic stains. This type of elastosis is typical of sun-damaged skin and the sun damage also accounts for the epithelial changes typical of actinic keratosis.

(c) Yes. Actinic keratosis and squamous cell carcinoma are known to be related to exposure to ultraviolet light. Therefore, an outdoor occupation or employment in a sunny climate are both important features in the patient's history.

11 (a) This is a lateral oblique radiograph showing a large radiopaque mass. It is not possible on this view alone to localise the site of the lesion.

(b) This is a submandibular sialogram. The main duct appears normal (submandibular ducts are considerably larger than parotid ducts). As the duct travels around the posterior border of the mylohyoid muscle it goes past the radiopacity and delineates a very atrophic and probably fibrosed submandibular gland.

(c) Yes, a scintiscan with technetium pertechnetate would demonstrate whether there was any remaining gland function. If the gland was not functioning then it should be removed as it will become infected. There is some evidence from scintiscanning studies that submandibular glands do regain function following removal of such calculi. In this case, surgical removal via an intraoral approach would be technically extremely difficult.

(d) If the calculus continues to produce symptoms then surgical removal of the gland is probably the best option. This patient declined surgery.

12 (a) This is a computerised tomographic (CT) scan taken at the level of the parotid glands.

(b) On the left side a sialogram has been undertaken simultaneously with the CT scan. Large areas of the gland do not fill.

(c) There are multiple cystic lesions within both parotid glands. The right parotid gland has one particularly large cystic area. The density scale shown on the left shows that these cystic areas have the density of fluid and are not solid. This is important to determine, because in HIV-positive patients there may be other reasons for persistent parotid enlargement, such as Kaposi's sarcoma or lymphoma.

(d) Fine needle aspiration of these cystic areas (guided by CT) drains them and they rarely reform. The cause of these lesions in HIV-positive patients is not clear.

13 (a) The relationship of the adjacent teeth raises suspicion of a pathological process that has displaced the canine tooth. Preoperative radiographs would help to evaluate this. These radiographs showed no bony pathosis.

(b) Fibrous epulis, giant cell lesion, pyogenic granuloma.

(c) The upper surface of the lesion is ulcerated, which might account for the occasional pain. This ulceration probably was a result of trauma.

(d) The photomicrograph shows an ulcerated surface overlying a highly cellular fibroblastic lesion. Bone formation is present in the deeper parts of the lesion. These features are typical of a fibrous epulis.

14 (a) This patient has relatively mild oral disease so topical therapy would probably be tried initially. Should this be unsuccessful then systemic steroids or griseofulvin or, rarely, cyclosporin A may be beneficial. The well-known nephrotoxicity of cyclosporin A precludes its use in this case; low-dose systemic prednisolone (e.g. 10 mg, preferably on alternate days) may be helpful. Griseofulvin has a role, particularly in women beyond child-bearing age. Monitoring of liver function and blood pressure would be required and therapy would need to be prolonged. In younger women, griseofulvin may interfere with the efficacy of oral contraceptive therapy. There have been claims also for the value of systemic retinoid therapy in erosive lichen planus.

(b) Epidemiological data suggest that most patients have two forms of the disease at any one time.

(c) Probably unlikely. Topical steroids (e.g. fluocinonide) under occlusion with an extended soft bite guard are effective and without systemic side effects.

15 (a) Fordyce spots.

(b) No.

(c) Yes. The features are those of a normal sebaceous gland.

16 (a) This is a denture-induced fibrous overgrowth.

(b) This patient really must wear a partial denture, as the lesion results from chronic irritation and the lesion grows backwards beneath the upper partial denture.

(c) It is occasionally appropriate to leave the upper denture out for a period of time, because the lesion will regress in size but it is unlikely to regress completely. Surgical excision is the best option followed by the provision of a new well-fitting partial denture.

17 (a) The white coloration to the base of this ulcer is due to fibrin deposition.

(b) Major aphthae contribute about 10% of aphthous ulceration. Minor aphthae account for about 80%, with herpetiform aphthae accounting for about 10% of ulceration.

(c) Aphthous ulceration has no proven relationship to infection but, nevertheless, topical tetracycline therapy is beneficial. The reason for this is unclear but several double-blind studies have shown the benefit of topical tetracycline therapy used as a mouthwash, particularly in major aphthae. It would appear also that the structure of tetracycline can be altered such that it no longer has antibiotic properties but will still enhance healing in aphthous ulceration, suggesting some other property of the drug has been important, perhaps an effect on protein turnover and wound healing.

18 (a) Although the division is not absolute the oral lesions of pemphigus vulgaris tend to be very painful, whereas the oral lesions of mucous membrane pemphigoid, although extensive, tend to be considerably less painful. This patient clearly has massive areas of ulceration with a fibrin base and erythematous margin and the relatively

ANSWERS

painless nature is highly suggestive of mucous membrane pemphigoid although immunofluorescence studies would be required to definitively separate the two.

(b) Drugs most likely to be used in treating this condition include systemic corticosteroid therapy, azothioprine and dapsone. A number of other drugs, including gold and methotrexate, have been used.

(c) Mucous membrane pemphigoid is not considered a lifelong disease although it is not clear whether patients actually go into long-term remission rather than actually be cured of their condition. Certainly lifelong review would be advisable.

19   (a) The linear nature of this lesion on the lateral margin of the tongue is highly suggestive of self-inflicted lesions. Some of the margins are hyperkeratotic, which also suggests similar injury previously in the same area.

(b) Blood tests are appropriate to rule out haematinic deficiency states or blood dyscrasias.

(c) This patient should be referred for a psychiatric opinion.

20   These lesions could be the result of a chemical burn from a denture-cleaning fluid or an unusual form of candidiasis or represent the early stages of a vesiculobullous disorder. History would exclude irritation from denture-cleansing agents; swabs and smears would exclude candidal infection, and direct immunofluorescence would be warranted to exclude a vesiculobullous disorder.

21   (a) This is Kaposi's sarcoma of the palate. In the earliest stages of Kaposi's sarcoma solitary or multiple areas of purplish lesions are evident as in this example.

(b) The condition is malignant in the sense that it can grow and extend locally and be locally invasive. Metastasis is uncommon, but multiple tumours occur.

(c) In a patient of this age group with Kaposi's sarcoma, HIV infection is highly likely and, by definition, the patient would therefore probably have AIDS. From the history other causes of immunosuppression, such as a renal transplant or a liver transplant, would be excluded.

22   (a) Age alone does not exclude oral squamous cell carcinoma and cases have been reported in very young children. The clinical appearance of this lesion at this site is highly suggestive of squamous cell carcinoma.

(b) Retinoid therapy is not effective treatment for invasive cancer but does play a role in potentially malignant lesions.

(c) If the lesion is dysplastic but not frankly invasive then systemic retinoids are an option but patients need to be monitored in view of their cholesterol and elevated blood lipids as a consequence of retinoid therapy.

23   (a) These are red blood cells.

(b) They have been stained with Giemsa stain.

(c) They are normal because they are of uniform size, shape and staining pattern.

24   (a) Two cell types are shown in this stain preparation. There are red blood cells with one neutrophil present.

90

(b) The abnormality shown, in contrast to **23**, is that the cells are much less densely stained (i.e. they are hypochromic). There is also more variation in cell size, with smaller cells being present. This is termed a microcytic blood picture.

(c) These features are typical of established iron deficiency anaemia.

25 (a) This is hairy leukoplakia. Its typical site of occurrence is the lateral margin of the tongue; it appears clinically as vertical striations along the lateral margin.

(b) The lesion is known to be caused by Epstein–Barr virus although there were also suggestions, in the earlier literature, of involvement of *Candida* and human papilloma virus. Patients do not usually seek treatment for hairy leukoplakia but, because Epstein–Barr virus belongs to the herpes group of viruses, it does respond to systemic acyclovir, albeit in high doses of between 2 and 3 g daily. Occasionally such lesions recur following treatment. As the condition is not potentially malignant, treatment is usually for cosmetic reasons and it can cause some cosmetic distress to patients if it extends towards the anterior margin of the tongue.

26 (a) This patient has pericoronitis. The condition classically arises around a partially erupted wisdom tooth that still has an operculum overlying at least part of the tooth. The inability to maintain good oral hygiene around the area encourages plaque and usually swelling of the operculum, which may be traumatised by the opposing tooth. Treatment would include local cleaning of the area with perhaps also occlusal adjustment of the opposing tooth. Metronidazole treatment is frequently prescribed although it is of unproven benefit.

(b) This patient presented with this pericoronitis but the condition was highly suggestive of having an underlying immune deficit because of the marked absence of an associated inflammatory response. This patient was counselled about HIV infection and was proven to be HIV positive, with the pericoronitis being the presenting feature of his disease.

27 (a) *Candida* species may be isolated from this lesion, which is erythematous candidiasis. The majority of *Candida* in this infection are actually present on the prosthesis or denture, with relatively small numbers of *Candida* within the lesion itself.

(b) The lesion appears red as a result of the low pH associated with candidal growth and also with the toxins in other mucosal irritant factors, which *Candida* produces.

28 The oral lesions associated in some patients with ulcerative colitis are known as pyostomatitis vegetans. These lesions are typically cobbled, may be extremely exuberant in appearance and are characterised by a rancid odour, not unlike that of necrotising ulcerative periodontitis.

29 (a) This patient has shingles, or herpes zoster infection, of the left intraorbital nerve. The patient has already been hospitalised, which seems wise with infections at this site because of the risk of cavernous sinus thrombosis.

(b) High-dose systemic acyclovir therapy is warranted, probably for a 10-day period.

(c) One important sequela of varicella zoster infection is post-herpetic neuralgia, which is difficult to treat. It has been suggested that a 10-day course of acyclovir may limit the development of this condition.

30   (a) These are rheumatoid nodules typical of rheumatoid arthritis.
(b) The salivary disease they are most typically associated with is secondary Sjögren's syndrome.

31   (a) This is erosive lichen planus of the lip. Most of the lower lip appears to have a white appearance typical of lichen planus, but there are localised areas of ulceration.
(b) The condition is difficult to treat: successful treatment may involve the use of systemic steroids.
(c) Lichen planus of the lip is not potentially malignant.

32   (a) Pyogenic granuloma, gingival hyperplasia, peripheral giant cell lesion and hyperparathyroidism.
(b) Pyogenic granuloma because the lesion is localised, inflammatory and has an ulcerated surface.
(c) Occlusion may play a significant role. The surface is ulcerated in some areas and hyperkeratotic in one area (the patient's right). This suggests a combination of acute and chronic trauma, probably occlusal in origin. The patient had a very deep overbite.
(d) The base of the lesion was incompletely removed and still in occlusion.
(e) Possible pressure resorption from the base of the lesion and the patient's lack of plaque control.

33   (a) This patient has symblepharon associated with mucous membrane pemphigoid. Areas of scarring are evident in the lower fornix.
(b) The oral condition associated with this is mucous membrane pemphigoid.

34   (a) No. Patients often think that oral lesions have been present for a much shorter time than they actually have. In some patients this is due to denial of any abnormality whilst others may genuinely not notice them until they reach a particular size or cause symptoms.
(b) The lesion is not epithelial – the epithelium looks normal and has no other features of a squamous cell papilloma.
(c) First thing in the morning when glycaemic control would be optimal, following insulin injection and a normal breakfast.
(d) The lesion could be arising from any submucosal tissue, i.e. nerves, muscles or adipose tissue. In this patient the lesion was an unusual lipoma.

35   (a) This lesion is somewhat elevated and does not have the characteristic appearance of a squamous cell papilloma. In addition, more distally there is another less-elevated lesion and overall the features are highly suggestive of malignancy.
(b) Biopsy is certainly indicated. Candidal leukoplakia would occur commonly at

this site, but the fact that the lesion is candidal leukoplakia and is elevated suggests it may already have progressed to a malignant state.

36   (a) No. There is no known relationship between epulides and iron deficiency.
(b) Peripheral giant cell granuloma, brown tumour of hyperparathyroidism, or possible pyogenic granuloma.
(c) If a giant cell lesion within bone is suspected, then serum calcium, phosphate and alkaline phosphatase and parathyroid hormone assay are indicated. Additional radiographs of the hands may show multiple radiolucencies in the phalanges, suggestive of osteitis fibrosis cystica.

37   (a) The lesion is clearly subepithelial and, therefore, could arise from any submucosal tissue in this area, such as minor salivary gland, muscle, adipose tissue or nerve. A vascular origin is unlikely given the colour of the lesion. The long duration of the lesion, yet without mucosal invasion, suggests it is benign.
(b) Minor salivary gland neoplasm. The lesion appears lobulated and is not the typical colour for a lipoma. About 50% of minor salivary gland neoplasms are malignant and 50% benign. This is unlike major salivary gland tumours where approximately 90% in the parotid are benign and approximately 70% of submandibular tumours are benign. The major salivary gland exception is the sublingual gland in which neoplasms are almost always malignant.
(c) Histological review reveals an epithelial neoplasm in which obvious duct differentiation is noted. Many of the ducts clearly have two layers of cells, the inner glandular layer and the outer myoepithelial layer. The tumour appears well circumscribed with no evidence of infiltration. This suggests that the lesion is a benign neoplasm and that conclusion is supported by the lack of cytological abnormality.
(d) This is a salivary adenoma, which in different areas shows a variety of patterns. The definitive diagnosis is a pleomorphic adenoma.

38   (a) Reactive melanosis due to smoking, physiological pigmentation or endocrinopathy, such as Addison's disease or Nelson's syndrome.
(b) Addison's disease is highly unlikely for two reasons. First, the patient is being treated for hypertension, and Addison's disease patients are classically hypotensive. Second, in Addison's disease there is typically a sodium-losing state, or hyponatraemia, but this patient's electrolytes are normal.
(c) No. Although the patient described the lesions as 'bruises', thus raising suspicion of a bleeding diathesis, the oral lesions do not in any way resemble purpura. Furthermore, they are bilaterally symmetrical, which also makes thrombocytopenia highly unlikely.
(d) Yes. Oral pigmentation has been reported in HIV-positive patients undergoing zidovudine (AZT) therapy; the oral mucosa, nails and skin can all be pigmented. It is also well recognised that there is an increased incidence of autoimmune disorders, such as Addison's disease, in HIV-positive patients.
(e) The cheek epithelium shows keratosis with no epithelial dysplasia. In the lamina propria, there are numerous brown pigment-laden cells. The pigment is melanin,

which is contained within macrophages. This is known as pigmentary incontinence, and the pigment is derived from melanocytes in the basal layers of the epithelium. Some basal keratinocytes also show melanin pigmentation, but this is less easily seen in this type of preparation.

39 (a) Yes. This patient has a very high exposure to cigarettes and the lesion is likely to be related to her smoking habit.

(b) Two factors are important in terms of the patient's age. First, she started smoking as a teenager. Smoking is an increasing problem in this age group and is giving rise to grave concern about the long-term health of the cohort, both in terms of cardiovascular disease and oral malignancy. The male:female ratio for oral malignancy has changed in the past 50 years from around 5:1 to nearer 1:1 (actually 1.8:1). The second concern is that, although she is still a young woman, she has had a high smoking intake for about 20 years. There certainly appears to be a wide range of susceptibility to leukoplakia, and indeed oral cancer, among individuals. Some individuals seem to be able to smoke 30 cigarettes a day for 50 years with no adverse oral consequences, yet others smoke lesser amounts or the same amount for reduced periods of time and do suffer serious or potentially serious oral consequences. Oral changes of this severity in a woman of this age group, who does not drink and is haematinically normal, give rise to considerable concern about her long-term prognosis.

(c) The histological features are likely to show epithelial dysplasia. A repeat biopsy after 3 months would be helpful to assess the biological progression of the lesion. (e.g. does it remain moderately dysplastic or progress to severe dysplasia?). Progression to severe dysplasia would warrant complete surgical excision. If the lesion remains moderately dysplastic then, clearly, cessation of the patient's smoking habit would be the best option. Advice about nicotine patch therapy would be helpful, as would hypnotherapy. Even extensive lesions such as this can clinically regress completely and be histologically normal. Other treatment options include laser surgery, topical bleomycin or systemic retinoids.

(d) Systemic retinoids and topical bleomycin are non-invasive treatment options. If the patient continues to smoke then neither option would be ideal. If the decision were made to prescribe retinoids, which are basically analogues of vitamin A known to affect epithelial maturation, then several precautions are required. Blood tests for cholesterol and lipids would be useful prior to retinoid therapy because both can become elevated with treatment. In a woman of this age group the principal concern has to be the teratogenicity of retinoids, which is very serious and affects all babies of pregnant women taking systemic retinoids. The patient would have to sign a disclaimer to this effect and agree not to become pregnant for 6 months following cessation of retinoid therapy. With this proviso, a daily systemic dose of 1 mg/kg/day is claimed to produce clinical resolution in approximately 60% of cases. Recurrence is possible on cessation of drug therapy.

40 (a) A right submandibular sialogram.

(b) Contrast media has been introduced into the duct to outline the ductal anatomy. The very marked radiopacity of the dye indicates an oil-based medium has been used. The gland is also overfilled and most gland detail is lost.

(c) The submandibular gland has ruptured, spilling the dye into the fascial planes of the neck. The prior irradiation had probably weakened the gland and overfilling has caused gland damage.

(d) Provided that infection does not supervene, the dye will be dispersed with time although this will take many months. The gland is unlikely to recover and is probably best removed surgically.

41 (a) This is a basal cell carcinoma. Usually the lesions are solitary and elevated. This lesion, in addition to the central elevated area, also has extended in a linear fashion laterally.

(b) Surgical excision. Basal cell carcinomas are relatively resistant to radiotherapy.

(c) No. For reasons that are not clear, basal cell carcinomas usually occur on the midface region.

42 (a) No. It is relatively rare to see oral candidiasis affecting the buccal mucosa. Exceptions to this are candidal leukoplakia and pseudomembranous candidiasis, usually as part of widespread candidiasis. Similarly, erythematous candidiasis can affect the buccal mucosa, usually in immunocompromised patients. This lesion appears uniform in colour and is neither erythematous nor speckled.

(b) The histological specimen shows a mildly atrophic epithelium overlying a mass of moderately dense collagenous connective tissue. The features are those of a simple fibrous overgrowth.

43 (a) Highly unlikely. Candidiasis rarely affects the lower alveolar region. The systemic antifungal therapy was principally for her palatal candidiasis.

(b) Extensive epithelial overgrowth arising from the surface and penetrating the underlying tissues was seen at low power in the microscopic sections. The high-power view, shown in the photomicrograph, clearly indicates the cytological features of malignancy and the diagnosis was of a squamous cell carcinoma.

44 (a) Reticular lichen planus, with interspersed red areas suggesting some areas of atrophy.

(b) The age group affected is normally the over-50 age group, with the condition being slightly more common in women in the over-50 age group.

(c) Epidemiological studies suggest that any one patient has at least two forms of the condition present at any one time, as in this case.

45 (a) The three abnormalities present are fissured tongue, angular cheilitis and white plaques on the dorsum of the tongue.

(b) The white plaques and angular cheilitis are both caused by candidal infection. The simultaneous occurrence of both oral lesions and nail-bed lesions is highly suggestive of systemic candidiasis.

ANSWERS

(c) The patient is suffering from one of the chronic mucocutaneous candidal syndromes. Several of these syndromes are linked to endrocrine abnormalities and referral to a physician is warranted. It is not inconceivable that adult HIV patients may present in this way and children with inherited immune defects may also present similarly.

46 (a) No, but a malignant neoplastic process is highly unlikely to be only this size after 10 years. Clinically there is no evidence of malignancy – the epithelium appears normal with no ulceration.

(b) The lesion is pedunculated because it is thought that denture trauma and movement create a hyperplastic epithelial response, which can only grow under the denture and thus is flattened and pedunculated.

(c) 'Leaf fibroma.' This is really an area of denture hyperplasia in the palate beneath a denture.

(d) Probably not. The lesion has no known drug association or relationship to smoking or alcohol. If rheumatoid arthritis was part of Sjögren's syndrome then reduced saliva may have exacerbated localised denture trauma. Conceivably, rheumatic involvement of the temporomandibular joint could make denture control difficult and also predispose to trauma.

47 (a) This lesion may be arising from the maxillary antrum. For this reason a posteroanterior sinus view would be worthwhile. In addition, an intraoral radiograph of the lesion would help identify any local pathosis, such as a retained root.

(b) This patient requires steroid cover for the biopsy procedure. This would either be in the form of a doubling of the daily dose of oral prednisolone or by an intravenous injection of 200 mg of hydrocortisone hemisuccinate. It would be wise to measure the patient's blood pressure prior to administering steroid therapy in case the patient is already unknowingly hypertensive.

(c) Almost certainly the inhaler and oral corticosteroids would encourage oral candidiasis. It may not be possible to reduce the dose of systemic steroids, although pulmonary function secondary to emphysema should be monitored regularly to see if the systemic steroid dose could be reduced. Because 80% of inhaled corticosteroids remain in the oral cavity, their presence and effect can be reduced by a mouth rinse or gargle with water following inhaler use. Patients with emphysema often receive systemic antibiotic therapy periodically, which would also encourage oral candidiasis.

(d) Pyogenic granuloma, oroantral fistula with prolapse of the lining of the antrum, carcinoma of the maxillary antrum, peripheral giant cell granuloma.

48 (a) The area of palate exactly corresponding to that beneath the upper denture is inflamed.

(b) Erythematous candidiasis. It was previously known as chronic atrophic candidiasis or denture sore mouth.

(c) No.

(d) Candidiasis is often termed the 'disease of the diseased'. Many factors predispose to oral candidiasis, including haematinic deficiency states, diabetes mellitus, xerostomia, poor denture hygiene, high carbohydrate diet, antibiotic therapy, steroid therapy, extremes of age and immunosuppression.

49 (a) Griseofulvin is regarded as a systemic antifungal drug.
(b) The drug is normally used for the management of athlete's foot, which is a fungal infection between the toes. The drug has also been used successfully to treat oral conditions, particularly oral erosive lichen planus. The mechanism of this is still speculative but it is thought that, in an analogous manner to athlete's foot, it actually increases intraepithelial integrity and perhaps in some way toughens up the mucosa, making it less likely to break down following minor trauma. Studies in aphthous ulceration have also suggested that griseofulvin may be of some benefit. It needs to be borne in mind that liver function tests and full blood counts are mandatory when someone is receiving griseofulvin therapy and they should also be warned that oral contraceptive therapy may be reduced in efficacy because of the drug's potential effect on steroid metabolism and, therefore, other contraceptive measures may be necessary.

50 (a) Bone, liver and gastrointestinal tract. Isoenzyme studies are used to distinguish the three types.
(b) No. First, the patient is too young for Paget's disease and too old for fibrous dysplasia. Second, the blood parameters measured effectively exclude both diseases but this is not invariable, depending on disease activity.
(c) Peripheral giant cell lesion, fibromatosis or neurofibroma.
(d) The second premolar shows marked hypercementosis. The bone on both sides of the premolar is irregular and lacks a normal trabecular pattern.

51 (a) Cryotherapy uses gas, e.g. carbon dioxide, to freeze lesions. The gas is under pressure and when it reaches the tip of the probe it gives off latent heat of vaporisation. This cools the tip to about −60°C and the tissues to about −20°C, probably for several millimetres beneath the mucosa. One disadvantage is that it allows no histological confirmation of the provisional diagnosis.
(b) It probably reduced the size of the lesion but the surface has ulcerated and not healed after 4 weeks.
(c) The main mass of the lesion comprises numerous vascular spaces. The differential diagnosis lies between a haemangioma and a pyogenic granuloma. The original clinical presentation was indicative of a developmental lesion rather than a traumatic lesion and the diagnosis is therefore of haemangioma.
(d) Yes. There is some experimental evidence that oral precancerous lesions partially treated with cryotherapy can promote progression to carcinogenesis.

52 These red blood cells differ from the cases described in **23** and **24** inasmuch as they are of unusual size and also a varied shape, i.e. they demonstrate anisopoikilocytosis. They are almost certainly a result of vitamin B_{12} deficiency associated with the autoimmune disease of pernicious anaemia.

ANSWERS

53   (a) Inability to smile symmetrically, indicating a right facial nerve weakness.
(b) No.
(c) Provided there were no contraindications, high-dose prednisone therapy.

54   (a) This patient has a right-sided facial nerve palsy. It could be idiopathic as a result of Bell's palsy but might also be due to Ramsay-Hunt syndrome, which is caused by varicella zoster infection of the geniculate ganglion.
(b) When associated with varicella zoster infection, facial nerve palsy is termed Ramsay-Hunt syndrome.
(c) Other causes of facial nerve palsy include trauma, HIV infection, Lyme disease, Bell's palsy, multiple sclerosis and Guillain–Barré syndrome.

55   (a) Squamous cell carcinoma. With such a prolonged history of smoking and alcohol abuse this patient has over a 40-fold increased risk of oral cancer than the general population.
(b) At least two tests should be performed. A blood coagulation screen is essential in such an individual, who is almost certain to have severely compromised liver function. Advice should be sought from a consultant haematologist on how to correct any identifiable coagulation disorder and this is likely to include vitamin K therapy. Additionally, the patient's hepatitis B status should be checked and the haematology laboratory notified of the result for infection-control purposes.
(c) The epithelium shows striking dysplasia, with increased numbers of mitoses and mitoses superficially in the epithelium being obvious features. The dysplasia in the area illustrated would be categorised as severe. In other areas the dysplasia extended through the full thickness of the epithelium and the diagnosis of carcinoma-in-situ was appropriate. In further sections early invasive squamous cell carcinoma was found to be arising from the dysplastic epithelium.

56   (a) Around 5% of Caucasians and about 38% of people of colour have oral pigmentation. Oral hyperpigmentation is somewhat age related and appears to increase with age.
(b) Malignant melanoma. It is impossible to be certain clinically about the nature of localised areas of oral pigmentation. If there is any doubt an excision biopsy is warranted because oral malignant melanoma has such a poor prognosis.
(c) An amalgam tattoo. In this condition amalgam debris is inadvertently introduced submucosally because of accidental contact with the bur during amalgam removal. Amalgam is left in an extraction socket as the filling breaks up either during tooth extraction or impression techniques when a tooth heavily restored with amalgam is being prepared for a cast gold or porcelain crown.

57   (a) In this age group the patient's recurrent oral ulceration is likely to be aphthous in nature. The palate shows features of erythematous candidiasis with white areas in the vault of the palate.
(b) Probably for at least two reasons. First, without good denture hygiene candidal species adhere to the fitting surface of the denture. This adhesion is the first step

in the development of infection because it permits candidal replication. Second, covering of the oral mucosa may limit access of naturally occurring antifungal substances in saliva to that area of the mouth.

58   (a) The photomicrograph illustrates a recently ruptured bulla in the soft palate. This is most likely to be due to angina bullosa haemorrhagica.
(b) The lesion arises spontaneously or as a result of local trauma.
(c) Recurrence is likely, although the condition tends to burn itself out over a period of several years.

59   (a) This is leukoplakia on the ventral aspect of the tongue. At this site such lesions are also termed sublingual keratosis but this term should be abandoned.
(b) Leukoplakia, particularly at this site, is potentially malignant.
(c) Management options include excluding haematinic deficiency states and accompanying candidal infection, eliminating risk factors, such as smoking and alcohol, and more active treatment regimes, such as topical bleomycin therapy or systemic retinoids. Laser surgery is another option.

60   (a) Several areas of submucosal bleeding are demonstrated.
(b) The blood disorder most likely to be associated with submucosal bleeding is thrombocytopenia. This is a serious disorder that occurs in various forms but always necessitates urgent referral because of the short half-life of platelets, which is in the order of 10 days. Normally, patients have platelet counts in excess of 170×10^9/litre; this patient had a platelet count of less than 20,000.

61   This photograph has been taken to demonstrate multiple petechiae at the posterior aspect of the nape of the patient's neck. This is the site where her collar could rest and illustrates that even minor trauma can cause bleeding at such sites.

62   (a) The bluish colour suggests the lesion is vascular in origin. Placing a glass slide against the lesion in such cases usually produces a blanching effect.
(b) Vascular lesions can be much larger than they appear clinically and can bleed profusely during excision. A preoperative assessment of the patient's platelet count would be wise. In addition, gadolinium scans are helpful in determining the extent of vascular malformations preoperatively.
(c) No, but in view of the patient's age and drug therapy, excision under local anaesthesia is much preferable to the risks of general anaesthesia.

63   (a) These are foliate papillae on the distal lateral margin of the tongue. They are part of the oropharyngeal glands, including the tonsil and the ring of Waldeyer.
(b) No, these lymphoid tissue aggregates are entirely normal and are usually noticed by patients either on examining their tongue or when they may enlarge following upper respiratory tract infections.
(c) No treatment is necessary but patients need to be reassured as to the benign nature of the condition.

64   (a) Squamous cell carcinoma. This is a classical site for such lesions, which are typically slow growing and painless.
(b) There are extensive downgrowths of epithelium, which are moderately dysplastic in parts. At first glance there does not appear to be invasion, but the epithelium is lying between muscle bundles and this is actually invasion. The diagnosis is of well-differentiated squamous cell carcinoma.
(c) Radiotherapy is highly effective in squamous cell carcinomas of the lip. Remarkably, even much more extensive lesions than this heal almost completely and without scarring. Surgical excision using a wedge excision is also effective but more invasive.
(d) Excellent. This clinically is a T1 N0 M0 lesion and survival at 5 years should be around 90–95%.

65   (a) Many chronic oral mucosal lesions are painless and are often detected on routine dental examination, as was the case here. If the patient was a regular dental attender (e.g. every 6 months) then it would be possible to put some kind of time scale to the evolution of the lesions. This is clearly not possible with irregular dental attenders.
(b) No. Together they are more than additive. There are about 200 potential carcinogens in tobacco, including some radioactive elements. Direct mucosal damage, perhaps influenced also by heat trauma, would be aided by the solvent action of alcohol, allowing penetration through the oral mucosa.
(c) This is a contentious area. Historically, 'dental sepsis' was thought to play a role in oral cancer. However, dental sepsis was also at that time implicated in a large number of systemic problems without scientific justification. One large study in China has, however, linked dental disease with oral cancer. It may be that individuals with poor oral dental care may also be those inclined to expose themselves to other risk factors for oral cancer.
(d) Microscopic examination shows an atrophic epithelium with prominent keratosis. Mild epithelial dysplasia is present and there was also mild pigmentation of the deeper layers of the epithelium and mild pigmentary incontinence. These features are consistent with a smoker's keratosis.

66   (a) The short duration of these lesions and the fact that they have coalesced into irregular ulcers is highly suggestive of herpetiform ulceration.
(b) These lesions are more common in women than men. All other types of aphthous ulceration are equally common in men and women.

67   (a) These yellow deposits around both eyes are termed xanthelasma.
(b) These lesions are idiopathic in some patients but may be associated in others with elevated blood lipids.
(c) Blood tests to measure cholesterol and other fatty acids are indicated. Cholesterol and fatty acids are only elevated in a minority of patients with xanthelasma but increased levels require exclusion because of the known association of hypercholesterolaemia with cardiac disease.

68   (a) This patient has suffered from a neoplastic lesion on the lateral margin of the tongue. What is being viewed is a replacement skin graft in that area.

(b) The fact that the anterior and posterior margins of the lesion, and indeed the superior margin, occur in a straight line is highly suggestive of iatrogenic disease, namely replacement of a skin graft in that area, as usually pathoses do not occur in straight lines.

(c) The graft itself does not appear normal and there is a cleft in it along the midborder; in addition, the area also appears speckled as it has been colonised by candidal species, which is a not uncommon problem with skin grafts in the oral mucosa.

69   (a) Lymphangioma. Multiple fluid-filled lesions are evident, arising submucosally. The lesions themselves are painless but trauma can produce bleeding into the lesion(s), as seen here.

(b) Doing nothing is an option. These lesions are small and may become relatively smaller as the child grows. Cryosurgery is an option but can be followed by massive swelling post-treatment. Surgical excision of the larger lesions perhaps is another option, as is electrocautery and laser therapy, although the latter is best suited to mucosal lesions.

(c) Approximately 50% occur in the head and neck region.

(d) Most surveys indicate that the vast majority of lymphangiomas arise in the first decade of life.

70   (a) A childhood exanthem with systemic upset such as measles.

(b) Around 3 years of age

71   (a) Candidal leukoplakia. This is the classical site for the condition and is frequently bilateral.

(b) The patient must have initial commensal carriage of candidal organisms, is often a smoker (around 80% of such patients smoke) and is usually a non-secretor of blood group substances. Approximately 75% of the general population secrete blood group substances in their saliva but the reverse is true for patients with candidal leukoplakia, where approximately 70% are non-secretors. Being a non-secretor has been associated with susceptibility to a wide variety of infections, including cholera, bacterial meningitis and urinary tract infections in women. The mechanism for this is unclear.

(c) Stopping smoking is a useful first step in management. The argument about whether smoking causes the lesion initially and then the lesion is colonised by candidal organisms seems to have been answered by the second stage of management, namely systemic antifungal therapy with fluconazole. This drug is spectacularly effective in candidal leukoplakia, resolving the lesion in 2–3 weeks following 1 week of 50 mg daily therapy. This response is much greater than could be anticipated from studies of epithelial kinetics and argues for candidal organisms being of primary importance. The common association between candidal infections generally and haematinic deficiency states does not seem to apply to this chronic form of oral candidiasis as these patients are usually haematinically normal.

(d) Long-term follow-up is important because unless risk factors, such as smoking, are addressed and effective therapy given, transition to malignancy is a well-recognised risk.

72   (a) Orofacial granulomatosis (OFG). Crohn's disease is unlikely since that usually develops in patients with long-standing (i.e. more than 10 years) bowel symptoms. In the absence of a previous history of facial nerve palsy, Melkersson–Rosenthal (M–R) syndrome is excluded. Some would argue that all the symptoms of M–R syndrome (i.e. facial swelling, facial nerve palsy and fissured tongue) need not all be present for diagnosis and use the term incomplete M–R syndrome. Clinically, M–R syndrome appears to be OFG with Bell's palsy, which indeed may be coincidental. Other conditions such as cheilitis granulomatosa seem to be identical to OFG and do not warrant recognition as a separate disease entity. On histological grounds sarcoidosis would come into the differential diagnosis but clinically is very dissimilar to OFG.

(b) The patient's dietary habits are fundamental to OFG. This patient has a high intake of the two commonest allergens that precipitate OFG, namely benzoic acid (E210–219) in the soft drinks (and possibly beer) and cinnamonaldelyde in the curries. OFG has no strong HLA association, nor is it inherited.

(c) Positive RAST results are found in about 65% of patients with OFG. RAST measures circulating IgE levels to common allergens, such as house-dust mite, pollen and animal dander. The agents to which the patients are positive on a RAST test seem not important in terms of OFG, which is usually due to allergy to dyes, colourings, flavourings or preservatives. The positive RAST does, however, indicate an atopic diathesis – around 50% of OFG patients are atopic and this probably represents an increased immunoreactivity to environmental substances generally.

(d) In patients who avoid dietary allergens the prognosis is excellent. It can, however, take up to 9 months to resolve the clinical condition. Not all patients are allergic to foodstuffs; some are allergic to metals, such as nickel, which can be more difficult to avoid.

73   (a) This tumour is arising in the minor salivary glands of the palate. A much higher proportion of minor salivary gland tumours are malignant than in the major salivary glands and there is a 50 or 60% chance of such a lesion being malignant.

(b) The most frequent malignant neoplasm is adenoid cystic carcinoma.

(c) The prognosis varies with the degree of invasion. Perineural spread is a well-characterised feature of adenoid cystic carcinoma and affects the prognosis.

74   (a) The patient obviously has bruising, in this case spontaneously around the lip region on the right hand side and also intraorally.

(b) The patient needs immediate referral as she may have thrombocytopenia, perhaps drug induced, or due to leukaemia, aplastic anaemia or marrow fibrosis.

75 (a) These two slides demonstrate a patient's right facial appearance and also appearance of the right parotid sialogram. The facial appearance of chronic lesions around the angles of the mouth and also the erythematous regions around the face are typical of glue intoxication or solvent abuse.

(b) The sialographic features in a person of this young age are of multiple areas of sialectasis typical of chronic recurrent parotitis of childhood.

(c) The management of chronic recurrent parotitis of childhood involves either treating each course of bacterial infection with systemic antibiotics or treating for prolonged periods of time, usually several months, with systemic antibiotic therapy.

76 (a) Candidal leukoplakia, which is also known as *Candida*-associated leukoplakia or chronic hyperplastic candidiasis.

(b) Yes, if untreated a small proportion of these lesions will become malignant over a 10–15 year span.

(c) Three predisposing factors to this condition appear to be previous carriage of candidal species in the oral mucosa, smoking and secretor status, as a vast majority of such patients are non-secretors of blood group substances in saliva. The fact that this condition responds extremely promptly to systemic antifungal therapy with fluconazole suggest that the candidal infestation is the most significant feature of the condition, which may also be known as speckled leukoplakia and, as is shown here, is characterised by red areas interspersed with white areas.

77 (a) Approximately 80% of cases of candidal leukoplakia occur at this site. The lesion has red and white areas, suggestive of speckled leukoplakia (candidal leukoplakia, *Candida*-associated leukoplakia, chronic hyperplastic candidiasis). The lesion does not quite extend to the commissure region and, with a history of smoking, smokers' keratosis is another possibility. The lesion could also be a traumatic keratosis from chronic cheek biting.

(b) For the patient to develop *Candida*-associated angular cheilitis the source of *Candida* would have to be the oral cavity (i.e. the patient must have previously had a commensal carriage of candidal organism). This would also be a prerequisite for developing candidal leukoplakia.

(c) Yes, some studies have shown that up to 50% of patients with angular cheilitis are iron deficient. It is not known if iron deficiency predisposes to oral carriage of candidal species.

(d) The epithelium shows keratosis, with a thick orthokeratinised stratum corneum. The cellular layers are of approximately normal thickness and there is no epithelial dysplasia. A patchy non-specific chronic inflammatory cell infiltration is noted in the lamina propria.

(e) Keratosis without histological features of dysplasia is not of immediate concern. However, other studies suggest that any smoking-related oral lesion is potentially malignant and therefore needs both long-term review and rebiopsy.

78 (a) It is likely the patient has Bell's palsy, which is an idiopathic lower motor neurone palsy of the facial nerve. It could also be the initial presentation of

Melkersson–Rosenthal syndrome but no other features were present to suggest this. Occasionally, other conditions, such as HIV infection and Lyme disease, can produce facial nerve palsy. The rapidity of onset makes a relationship to a neoplastic process highly unlikely. There was also no oral or pharyngeal ulceration to suggest Ramsay-Hunt syndrome.

(b) Systemic prednisolone is the treatment of choice, although its efficacy is not proven. However, not treating the condition may lead to incomplete recovery and a resulting cosmetic and functional problem that may need plastic surgery. High-dose prednisolone, usually 40–60 mg daily, is needed for periods of up to 3 weeks. It is wise to measure blood pressure prior to prescribing such high doses of prednisolone and in the UK patients would be issued with a steroid warning card. This card should be retained by the patient for 2 years and steroid cover would be required during that time for dental extraction.

(c) The patient has developed steroid-induced acne. This is a relatively uncommon complication of such short-term therapy and was treated with systemic erythromycin.

(d) If patients with Bell's palsy have high-does prednisolone therapy commenced within a few days of onset of the condition then the prognosis is excellent. If the facial palsy is due to Ramsay-Hunt syndrome (which usually occurs in older subjects) the outcome is usually less favourable.

79   (a) Generally, the prognosis is worse in a patient who does not smoke or drink alcohol but develops an oral squamous cell carcinoma. The natural history of such primary lesions is often the patients develop multiple primary lesions and often the fourth or fifth new primary condition is clinically aggressive and results in death shortly thereafter. The reason for this relatively poor prognosis is not known.

(b) A TNM staging system is the normal system used. T = tumour size, N = regional lymph node involvement and M = presence or absence of distant metastases. Clearly larger lesions, local lymph node involvement and distant metastases worsen the prognosis.

(c) The overall 5-year survival from oral cancer is probably in the region of 40–50%, but this has wide regional variations. For example, over 90% of patients with lip cancers would be expected to survive at 5 years.

80   (a) This is erythematous candidiasis limited to certain areas of the hard palate and attached gingiva. The patient is clearly dentate and therefore would not have a partial denture.

(b) This lesion has developed in this dentate patient because of poor appliance hygiene, associated with an acrylic orthodontic retaining appliance.

81   This patient was admitted to hospital because of multiple dental abscesses and a diagnosis of glandular fever was made serologically. He also had some bruising beneath the right eye, which was caused by thrombocytopenia, a potentially serious side effect of glandular fever.

82   (a) Non-caseating epithelioid granuloma

(b) Sarcoidosis. About 6% of sarcoidosis patients have salivary gland involvement, which is usually bilateral and may cause some discomfort. Ocular involvement is not uncommon.

(c) Bilateral hilar lymphadenopathy. In addition to plain radiographs, magnetic resonance imaging (MRI) can be used to detect smaller sarcoid deposits.

(d) Serum angiotensin converting enzyme (SACE) levels may be helpful. SACE is produced by sarcoid granulomata and in a patient such as this, who clearly has systemic disease, SACE levels would be elevated.

(e) Generally, sarcoidosis is a self-limiting disease lasting 2–3 years. It can last longer in some patients. Assessment of pulmonary function and an ophthalmic opinion would be advised. Systemic corticosteroid therapy is the mainstay of treatment.

83   (a) This is minor recurrent aphthous ulceration.

(b) Deficiency states associated with it are iron, vitamin B_{12}, folic acid, vitamin B_1, vitamin B_2 and vitamin B_6.

(c) Management includes exclusion of deficiency states, identification of any allergic predisposing factors and attempts to manage stress, which can precipitate the disorder in some individuals. Symptomatic treatment ranges from topical to systemic steroids.

84   (a) If the lesion is unilateral at this site then it possibly is a lichenoid reaction, which tends to be more unilateral than bilateral.

(b) A biopsy may be useful in identifying a cause and any dysplasia present within a lesion.

(c) Adjacent amalgam restorations may be of relevance as they are involved in some oral lichenoid reactions. Such amalgams tend to be in place for more than 5 years and they tend to be associated with poor oral hygiene. The proximity of this lesion to fairly large amalgam restorations raises this possibility, which would have to be excluded by proper patch testing. Patients allergic to amalgam restorations are almost always allergic to the ammoniated mercury component of their amalgams.

85   The factors of main concern about this lesion are first, it is in a middle-aged to elderly person; second, it is elevated; and third, it is in the lateral margin of the tongue. All these features are highly suggestive of squamous cell carcinoma, which would need to be excluded on biopsy.

86   (a) Extensive bone loss is present in the region of the extracted teeth. The bone loss is irregular, greatly in excess of anything that could be due to dental disease and is highly suggestive of malignancy. In addition, there is a large well-delineated radiolucency further anteriorly. This is likely to be a residual cyst unrelated to the other radiological changes because it appears benign.

(b) Squamous cell carcinoma. The lesion is extensively infiltrative and, because it already has invaded bone, has a very poor prognosis.

(c) This is a case of an advanced, poorly differentiated squamous cell carcinoma in a young patient. The mucosa overlying the extraction sockets has not healed, some 5 weeks postoperatively, as a result of neoplasia. The bone pain from the tumour probably led to the teeth extraction in the first instance. Radical surgery of the mandible and neck lymph nodes, combined with radiotherapy, is the best management option but even then the 5-year survival is likely to be only about 15%. This patient only lived for 4 months after diagnosis.

87   (a) No. Edentulous patients with dentures are much more likely to have candidal organisms as the pathogenic species. In any case, this patient does not have clinical angular cheilitis but rather a hyperplastic nodular area of the right commissure without erythema, scaling or ulceration.

(b) Biotyping. This procedure, which depends on the results of sugar fermentation tests, can type individual species of *Candida*. In cases of angular cheilitis due to *Candida* the same biotype is isolated from the angles of the mouth (via an oral rinse). In an analogous way, phage typing can be used to identify staphylococcal species at the angles and from the anterior nares.

(c) Amyloidosis, but xanthogranuloma has a similar clinical appearance.

(d) Any chronic inflammatory condition can predispose to amyloidosis. In this case, what the patient described as 'rheumatism' was in fact rheumatoid arthritis, which had been present for many years. Amyloidosis is a known long-term complication of rheumatoid arthritis.

88   (a) This is doubtful. Certain forms of psoriasis, particularly guttate psoriasis, are asociated with an increased prevalence of geographic tongue. The histological appearances of psoriasis and geographic tongue do show some similarities.

(b) This is a result of keratosis, either as an intrinsic part of the lesion or from superimposed chronic trauma. Once saliva is absorbed into the keratin layers the optical properties of the epithelium are changed and the lesion appears white.

(c) The polypoid lesion is an area of fibrous overgrowth. This is covered by a heavily keratinised epithelium, which accounts for the white appearance in the mouth. The keratosis was due to frictional irritation.

(d) The biopsy of right buccal mucosa shows a poorly formed stratum corneum in an epithelium, which should normally be non-keratinised. This appearance is due to frictional irritation and may have been caused by cheek biting.

89   (a) No. Although haemangiomata can occur anywhere they are exceedingly rare on the gingivae.

(b) Clinically, preoperative radiographs are probably not necessary but medico-legally they should have been undertaken. It is conceivable that the lesion has arisen from bone and extended buccally.

90   (a) Minor, major and herpetiform. The clinical distinction between each is largely on the basis of time to healing and ulcer behaviour. Thus, major aphthae take more than 3 weeks to heal whereas minor aphthae heal in less time than this. Both major and minor aphthae remain as solitary or multiple ulcers whereas herpetiform aphthae coalesce. Aphthous type ulceration is also a feature of Behçet's disease, orofacial granulomatosis and HIV infection.

(b) Recognised haematinic deficiency states associated with aphthae include iron, vitamin B_{12} folic acid, vitamin B_1, vitamin B_2 and vitamin B_6. Often such deficiencies require investigation. Replacement therapy is usually effective in the treatment of aphthae.

91   (a) There were two main reasons. First, the appearance of the buccal mucosa does not suggest a traumatic lesion and there are also some associated erythema – often considered a clinical feature of some concern in potentially malignant oral lesions. Secondly, with a history of difficulty with complete dentures it is likely that the alveolar lesion is traumatic. Moreover, the alveolar ridge is naturally keratinized while the buccal mucosa is not. When clinical doubt exists, however, it would be entirely appropriate to biopsy both sites.

(b) Yes. This would be mandatory in view of her previous history of rheumatic heart disease. Infective endocarditis still has a high mortality – about 50% – and, therefore, antibiotic cover is obligatory in this case.

(c) The epithelium is heavily keratinised and the viable cellular layers are atrophic. Some slight irregularity of the basal cells is present, amounting to minimal epithelial dysplasia.

92   Sialosis is defined as a non-inflammatory, non-neoplastic, persistent enlargement of the salivary glands, usually the parotid glands. The condition is associated with altered liver function, undiagnosed maturity-onset diabetes, some drug therapy, acromegaly and anorexia nervosa. Some cases appear idiopathic.

93   (a) The lesion is of prognostic significance as a proportion of patients who have hairy leukoplakia go on to develop AIDS within the next 2 years.

(b) Hairy leukoplakia is not pathognomonic of HIV infection and has been described in a number of other patients with immune deficiency from a variety of causes, usually from drug therapy following renal or liver transplantation.

94   (a) Denture-induced hyperplasia. This is an uncommon site for this condition. However, the clinical appearance, the history of previous excision, the age of the dentures and the denture-wearing pattern are all highly suggestive of denture-induced hyperplasia. The surface of the lesion has ulcerated.

(b) The main histological feature is a mass of dense fibrous tissue. The superficial connective tissues and the overlying epithelium show non-specific inflammatory changes.

(c) The denture issue would need to be addressed. Complete dentures should normally be replaced every 5 years. During those years bony remodelling will have

ANSWERS

taken place and the denture will not fit as well as previously. Consequently, movement of the dentures would cause irritation and a hyperplastic epithelial response. Wearing the dentures only during the day would also be helpful.

95 (a) The main danger to a doctor from venepuncture is inadvertent needlestick injury. Transmission of hepatitis B is possible and also transmission of HIV infection, although this is less likely.
(b) This region of the arm is called the antecubital fossa.
(c) No, haemophiliacs do not bleed excessively following venepuncture as they have a normal blood vessel wall structure and also normal platelet function, which are the two main factors that limit bleeding following venepuncture.

96 (a) The medical condition that made this patient's condition worse is the state of being atopic. Atopy predisposes to severe forms of primary herpetic gingivo-stomatitis, a condition known as Kaposi's varicelliform eruption.
(b) An individual in the early stages of the disease requires medical therapy, with hospitalisation and adequate fluid intake. Systemic acyclovir is also warranted.

97 (a) This patient has multiple vesicular lesions at the vermilion junction of the lip. The condition is typical of recurrent herpes labialis.
(b) The condition is infective as it is usually caused by herpes simplex type 1.
(c) Its recurrence is caused by a variety of factors, including exposure to sunlight, cold, menstruation, trauma and stress.

98 (a) Bony sequestrum, which has caused reactions of the overlying epithelium.
(b) Hopefully not. Proper radiological protection guidelines should safeguard radiographers from occupational ionising radiation. Such sequestrae do occur in apparently healthy subjects with no history of exposure to ionising radiation.

99 (a) Microscopic examination shows non-specific chronic ulceration, with a vigorous granulation tissue response in the base of the ulcer. There is also an area of stratified squamous epithelium beneath the base of the ulcer. This is due to squamous metaplasia of a minor salivary gland duct. Note the normal minor salivary gland ducts adjacent to this metaplastic area. It may be necessary for the pathologist to take multiple sections to confirm the nature of such metaplastic epithelium, in order that an erroneous diagnosis of an invasive neoplasm is not made.
(b) As in **6**, there is chronic non-specific ulceration in an elderly patient. Diabetes mellitus is known to cause a vasculopathy and perhaps this may be involved in the pathogenesis of the lesion but this is unproven.
(c) Possibly, but it is an unusual site. Normally, self-inflicted lesions are on the face or in the anterior region of the mouth. The patient suffered from depression but patients who deliberately self inflict injury on themselves, whilst clearly not psychologically normal, rarely produce such lesions. Further evidence of the lack of a relationship between depression and self-inflicted injury is that whilst depressed patients do not infrequently commit suicide, suicide is very rare in patients who deliberately mutilate themselves.

100 (a) This is a lateral view of a parotid sialogram.
(b) There is obvious sialectasis present. The patient is in his late teens. The two most likely diagnoses are chronic recurrent parotitis of childhood (CRPC) or Sjögren's syndrome. The patient is a little old for CRPC although the sialectasis associated with this condition may persist until around age 30 years. On the other hand, the patient is a little young for Sjögren's syndrome. The clinical history, probably coupled with a labial gland biopsy, should allow a definitive diagnosis.
(c) Sialectasis arises when the contrast medium enters the duct system and passes out between the ductal cells, accumulating periductally. In two-dimensional radiographs this gives the appearance of sialectasis.

101 (a) A salivary scintiscan in an anteroposterior direction.
(b) The patient's left parotid gland shows uptake, as do both submandibular glands. Some isotope has already entered the mouth, as seen in the centre. The patient's right parotid gland is non-functioning.
(c) As the parotid gland has no function it will be subject to repeated ascending bacterial infection from the mouth. Surgical removal of the gland is one option but is likely to be surgically difficult because of the number of previous episodes of infection causing fibrosis. Duct ligation is another option and was undertaken in this case. In an effort to eliminate any residual infection within the gland antibiotics may be injected in a retrograde manner into the duct prior to ligation.

102 (a) Yes. The lesion has some features that could be considered consistent with submucosal bleeding and, thus, thrombocytopenia is worth excluding. However, if the lesion had genuinely been present for 6 months then an acquired blood dyscrasia is unlikely.
(b) An atrophic epithelium overlies connective tissue containing numerous dilated vascular spaces. These spaces do not contain blood. The appearance is of a vascular hamartoma and, since the spaces do not contain blood, the most likely diagnosis is a cavernous lymphangioma.

103 (a) There are three lesions evident on this clinical photograph. The area in the centre is obviously elevated and is a squamous cell carcinoma, proven by a biopsy.
(b) The most clinically significant features of oral carcinoma, apart from ulceration, are that the lesion is elevated and appears on the lateral margin of the tongue.
(c) Both the anterior and indeed posterior lesions signify field change as it is recognised that, even though other areas of the oral mucosa are not carcinomas at presentation, they are not biologically normal either. This squamous cell carcinoma developed in a patient who did not smoke or drink.

104 The nature of these lesions are highly suggestive of them being self-inflicted. Multiple areas of ulceration and scarring are present on the inner aspect of the upper lip. The inside of the upper lip is not a site that is particularly associated with any common oral diseases and what is highly suggestive of artefactual disease is the fact that there are several areas at different stages of healing. In addition, there are old scars from previous injury. These lesions are therefore artefactual and the patient requires referral for a psychiatric opinion. It is of some interest that although these patients self-inflict injury they are, in fact, at low risk from suicide.

105 (a) The differential diagnosis of this lesion may include a giant cell tumour, a pyogenic granuloma or lesions related to parathyroid disorders.
(b) Blood tests are appropriate to measure parathyroid hormone and also urea and electrolytes.
(c) Radiographs of the area itself may be helpful to determine any bony involvement and also radiographs of the hands may be useful in cases of osteitis fibrosis cystica.

106 Two pathological conditions associated with generalised pigmentation include Addison's disease and Nelson's syndrome.

107 (a) This investigation demonstrates the patches that are to be applied to the forearm during testing for type 1 hypersensitivity reactions, including orofacial granulomatosis. The patches are applied for a 20-minute period and then read clinically and, ideally, also thermographically.
(b) Patch testing is of value in a variety of orofacial diseases, including orofacial granulomatosis, some cases of minor aphthous stomatitis, lichenoid reactions thought to be due to dental materials, erythema multiforme, type 3 burning mouth syndrome and patients thought to be allergic to, or intolerant of, dental prostheses.

108 (a) This lesion apparently arose following minor trauma and what is worrying is the fact that there is extensive swelling with minimal erythema. The swelling is grossly out of proportion with what would be expected following minor trauma.
(b) Blood tests are appropriate to look for blood dyscrasias and in this patient Waldenström's hypergammaglobulinaemia was detected.
(c) In the first instance topical symptomatic treatment may be of benefit but clearly the patient requires urgent referral to a specialist unit.

109 (a) Mucocele.
(b) Mucoceles are usually due to mucus extravasation from damaged ducts. The extravasated mucus is surrounded by granulation tissue.
(c) Yes.

110 (a) Geographic tongue, also known as erythema migrans or benign migratory glossitis. It is a fallacy that this condition actually spreads round the tongue, and serial photographic studies suggest that the depapillated areas, which lack filiform papillae, begin in one area, gradually expand and then may contract to heal normally only to reappear some time shortly afterwards in an adjacent area.
(b) No, the condition is not inherited.
(c) The condition seems to be idiopathic, but in some cases is related to zinc deficiency. Systemic zinc replacement therapy over a 3-month period almost always

resolves a patient's symptoms of discomfort on eating and in 50% of cases it would be expected to make the oral mucosa clinically normal.

111 (a) Lichen planus. The patient appears to have reticular lesions but these are atypical. The left buccal mucosa is certainly lichenoid but the elevated nature of the lesion on the right buccal mucosa is not typical of lichen planus.
(b) Candidal leukoplakia. It is possible that this lesion was also being traumatised and this was giving rise to the discomfort. The best treatment option is surgical excision, as was performed here, but that was for diagnostic purposes. Usually such lesions are subject to an incisional biopsy first to confirm the diagnosis.
(c) Systemic antifungal therapy with fluconazole is known to be extremely effective in candidal leukoplakia with clinical resolution occurring in 2–3 weeks following daily (50 mg) therapy for 1 week. Only about 20% of patients with candidal leukoplakia do not smoke.

112 (a) Laugier–Hunziker syndrome.
(b) No.
(c) Once developed the pigmentation is thought to be permanent.

113 (a) This is erythematous candidiasis of the palate.
(b) Predisposing factors to candidiasis include blood dyscrasias, xerostomia, drug therapy with corticosteroids or antibiotics and a high carbohydrate diet. Immuno-deficiency states and poor denture hygiene may also be contributing factors.
(c) The fact the patient is diabetic is relevant as diabetics exhibit clinical candidiasis at a lower candidal load than non-diabetic subjects. It would appear that in diabetic patients there is a predilection for adhesion of candidal species to the oral mucosa.

114 (a) A parotid sialogram is being undertaken using an orthopantomogram (OPG).
(b) Using an OPG does not allow lateral and anteroposterior views. This is a disadvantage and it can be difficult to determine whether a lesion is in the parotid gland at all. Secondly, it is technically more difficult as the patient must be standing and, thirdly, there is considerable contralateral artefact.

115 A biopsy is the most useful way of determining between erosive lichen planus (LP) and discoid lupus erythematosus (DLE). Although these two conditions appear similar on biopsy there tends to be more vasculitic involvement with lupus erythematosus and a less pronounced subepithelial lymphocytic infiltrate.

116 (a) It is of some significance as to whether the lesion is of LP or DLE. DLE may occasionally develop into systemic lupus erythematosus (SLE), which has multiple manifestations, whereas LP is likely to remain as a localised disorder. There is also some suggestion that DLE may be potentially malignant and, although this question has also been raised in relation to LP, it seems to be a rare clinical event.
(b) Antinuclear factors may be helpful in a diagnosis. These would be negative in LP and would be unlikely to be positive in DLE but they would be expected to be positive if the patient develops SLE.

117 (a) It does not appear to obviously inflamed but low-grade periosteal lesions can arise frequently related to periapical infection.

(b) Yes. Periapical infection in the absence of obvious crown pathosis can occur with some developmental abnormalities of dentine.

118 (a) This condition is likely to be due to an amalgam tattoo. This follows the inadvertent introduction of particles of amalgam restorations beneath the epithelium, usually during tooth preparation or, occasionally, tooth extraction.

(b) A radiograph may be helpful in identifying amalgam particles beneath the epithelium although the odd clinical feature of amalgam tattoos is the fact that biopsy shows tiny fragments of amalgam present despite the intense clinical pigmentation.

(c) The main differential diagnosis of a deeply pigmented lesion of the oral mucosa is malignant melanoma. As both amalgam tattoos and malignant melanoma are painless in the early stages, excision biopsy is probably warranted to confirm the diagnosis when radiographs show no abnormality.

119 (a) In cyclic neutropenia there is a cyclical diminution in neutrophil count, usually over a 4-week period. Episodes of oral ulceration coincide with the lowest neutrophil counts. To confirm the diagnosis, blood is taken on consecutive weeks for about 6 weeks. The haematology laboratory is asked to provide a differential white cell count over the 6-week period. The neutrophil count is never normal but records very low levels at some stage during this sequential sampling, thus confirming the diagnosis.

(b) Periodontal disease is a well-recognised feature of cyclic neutropenia. Usually the pattern of bone loss is more marked in the lower incisors and first molar region and resembles juvenile periodontitis although, of course, the patient is much older.

120 (a) Pyogenic granuloma in this area may be precipitated by calculus or an inadequate cervical restoration or, indeed, the presence of a foreign body in a periodontal pocket, such as a toothbrush bristle.

(b) The rolled margin to the lesion would require squamous cell carcinoma to be included in the differential diagnosis and, indeed, this lesion is a biopsy-proven squamous cell carcinoma.

(c) A radiograph may be helpful to demonstrate intrabony involvement; however, in this instance, intraoral peripheral radiographs demonstrated no abnormality.

121 (a) This is median rhomboid glossitis, albeit a very extensive example.

(b) It is caused by *Candida albicans*, which appears to have a predilection for colonising the midline dorsum of the tongue in the posterior aspect. The condition is also twice as common in diabetics than in non-diabetics.

(c) The drug most likely to precipitate this condition is steroid-inhaler therapy. About 80% of inhaled steroids remain on the oral mucosa and their effect on the local immune response encourages candidal colonisation and infection. A mouth rinse following steroid inhaler therapy should minimise the retention of the drug in the oral cavity.

122   In this lesion the overlying mucosa appears largely normal although clearly it is elevated. These features suggest pathological changes in the underlying connective tissue and may involve neural tissue, muscle or even fat. The clinical appearance does not suggest either lymphangioma or an haemangioma.

123   (a) Such lesions have been called syphilitic leukoplakia and are usually associated with the tertiary stage of syphilis. It is not clear whether syphilis itself causes the lesions or whether the arsenicals that patients were treated with played a role.
(b) This patient obviously suffers from black hairy tongue and has an unusual lesion on the left lateral margin distally that resembles lichen planus.

124   (a) The presentation of a large malignant-looking ulcer in the palate preceded by paraesthesia is highly suggestive of necrotising sialometaplasia. This is a benign self-limiting condition thought to be due to infarction of minor salivary glands beneath the epithelium. It can be confused, both clinically and histologically, with squamous cell carcinoma and might be more frequent in pregnant women.
(b) The condition may be related to the dressed tooth because a local anaesthetic may have been given to allow treatment of that tooth. It has been suggested that vasoconstriction of the greater palatal vessels following local trauma precipitates infarction in minor salivary glands.

125   (a) These are mandibular tori, which in this patient are unusually large.
(b) Mandibular tori are associated both with temporomandibular disorders and migraine.

126   (a) Pus is seen emanating from the parotid duct orifice.
(b) Acute suppurative parotitis.
(c) Many organisms can be cultured from an aspirate of the main duct itself. The main organisms implicated are staphylococcal and streptococcal species but, increasingly, anaerobic organisms are also implicated.
(d) Parotid sialography. About 80% of patients who have had an episode of acute suppurative parotitis have a parotid gland abnormality. This is mainly due to mucous plugs, benign duct strictures or salivary calculi. In addition, Sjögren's syndrome can first present as acute suppurative parotitis.

127   (a) This is widespread nicotinic stomatitis of the palate and there are also white areas present on the dorsum of the tongue.
(b) Nicotinic stomatitis in itself is not potentially premalignant but the oral mucosa generally may be at risk from such a high tobacco intake.
(c) The condition is caused by the heat of smoking (usually pipe smoking) or the irritants present within tobacco.

128 (a) Biopsy of this lesion on the inner aspect of the lower alveolus is sometimes difficult and care would have to be taken to ensure that the lesion is dissected in such a way that primary closure is possible.

(b) Non-resorbable sutures are usually the treatment of choice because, although resorbable sutures do not need to be removed, they are considerably more uncomfortable in the mouth than non-resorbable sutures. In addition, there is an onus on patients who know that they have to have their sutures removed by the clinician to return for removal and also for discussion of the biopsy result. On occasion, the patients fail to attend for review when non-resorbable sutures are placed. This can present a management problem.

129 (a) The main features are of a diffuse white lesion extending along the gingival margin. In addition there is an atrophic area within this faint white area.

(b) Lichenoid reaction. As the lesion is unilateral it is more likely to be a lichenoid reaction than lichen planus.

(c) In both lichen planus and lichenoid reactions the inflammatory changes can lead to mucosal atrophy. It would be wise to exclude other causes of mucosal atrophy, e.g. iron deficiency. Another blood test that may be helpful is investigation of whether the patient has circulating basal cell cytoplasmic antibodies. These autoantibodies occur in a proportion of patients with drug-induced oral lichenoid reactions.

(d) The epithelium is atrophic and keratinised. In the upper lamina propria there is a diffuse infiltration of chronic inflammatory cells. Migration of lymphocytes into the epithelium is noted and the deeper cell layers of the epithelium appear to be being damaged by an immune reaction.

130 (a) These lesions are squamous cell papillomas.

(b) They are caused by one of the many types of human papilloma virus.

(c) The infection is likely to be indigenous and may have spread from some other site, such as the fingers, in this individual.

131 (a) These lesions are not erythroplakia because they are not homogeneous and they also include areas of fibrin within them, suggesting an ulcerative process that is attempting to heal. Erythroplakia itself is usually a homogeneous red area, described as having a velvety appearance.

(b) A biopsy of the lesion is indicated, along with haematinic investigations to exclude deficiency states. On the opposite site of the soft palate (the patient's left side) there are signs of scarring and it is not inconceivable that this is perhaps an early stage major aphthous ulceration.

132 (a) Yes, major aphthae tend to occur towards the posterior aspect of the mouth.

(b) Behçet's disease is partly determined on clinical grounds with the involvement of genital and ocular lesions but HLA status may also be of value in confirming the diagnosis.

133 (a) This patient has a squamous cell carcinoma arising in the undersurface of the right ventral aspect of the tongue.
(b) This patient's brother had the same condition. Oral squamous cell carcinoma is not familial but both brothers shared a habit of excessive smoking and alcohol intake so the similarity relates to social habits rather than genetic predisposition.

134 (a) These are bony exostoses.
(b) The lesions are not usually apparent on radiographs. This is probably because the cortical bone itself is normal and there is an increase in cancellous bone, which would not be evident on radiographs.
(c) Bone exostoses are associated with some syndromes, particularly Gardner's syndrome.

135 (a) This patient is undergoing sialography.
(b) The submandibular gland, in this case on the right side, is being investigated.
(c) The abnormality shown is a large calculus present within the duct system. The radiopaque contrast medium seemed to enter the duct system normally, pass distally round the posterior border of myelohyoid and there encounter a large calcified mass within the duct system. The dye, however, is able to pass round the calculus and enter the remaining aspects of the gland, which have been grossly atrophied as a result of chronic sialadenitis; very little of the original gland structure remains.

136 (a) Mucosal disorders that most commonly affect the hard palate are candidal infections beneath dentures and vesiculobullous disorders. This lesion is clearly ulcerated with a surface fibrin clot. It is not due to *Candida* and is likely to be due to one of the vesiculobullous disorders.
(b) The main differential diagnoses in this case would lie between pemphigus vulgaris and mucous membrane pemphigoid.
(c) The single most important laboratory investigation is direct immunofluorescence from a biopsy of non-ulcerated epithelium. In the case of pemphigus vulgaris this would demonstrate antibodies of IgG deposited in the intercellular cement region. In the case of mucous membrane pemphigoid it would demonstrate IgG deposition in a linear pattern at the basement membrane.

137 (a) The most common cause of oral pigmentation is racial or physiological. Such pigmentation usually occurs in the buccal mucosa and is symmetrical.
(b) Addison's disease can be excluded by performing a synacthen test. This involves measuring the adrenal response to an injection of synthetic ACTH and measuring both the baseline level of cortisol and the elevation. In true Addison's disease there would also be alterations in urea electrolytes, with a particularly high potassium value, and the patient may also be hypotensive.

138 (a) This is a squamous cell carcinoma arising in the buccal mucosa and extending on to the alveolar ridge and palate.

(b) Surgical excision may be successful in this case in eradicating the initial tumour but multiple primary tumours are well recognised to develop in patients with squamous cell carcinoma and the whole oral mucosa would need monitoring on a lifelong basis.

139 (a) This patient clearly has marked gingival hyperplasia. Causes for this could be cyclosporine-induced hyperplasia, phenytoin-induced hyperplasia and nifedipine-induced hyperplasia or gingival fibromatosis. Mouth breathing is sometimes a contributory factor and other cases appear idiopathic.

(b) The condition is thought to be more severe in the lower arch because of the difficulty in maintaining oral hygiene and the false pockets that form with the gingival overgrowth are exacerbated by poor oral hygiene.

140 (a) Lesions are evident on the soft palate and also the dorsum of the tongue. The clinical appearance is strongly suggestive of a lymphangioma, which is a hamartoma.

(b) Biopsy would be necessary to confirm the diagnosis but hospitalisation is advised as there is occasionally extensive swelling postoperatively.

141 (a) This patient has desquamative gingivitis.

(b) This condition is associated with lichen planus, pemphigus and mucous membrane pemphigoid, although clinically similar lesions can occur in orofacial granulomatosis.

(c) If the lesions are due to desquamative gingivitis associated with lichen planus, pemphigus or mucous membrane pemphigoid then topical steroid therapy under occlusion and in an extended soft appliance is warranted. Studies suggest that the 5-minute application, morning and night, of topical fluorinated steroids is not associated with significant immunosuppression but does result in resolution of the condition.

142 (a) The abnormality shown is a scalloped appearance to the anterior tip of the tongue.

(b) The condition has been caused by a chronic habit of forcing the tongue between the natural dentition.

(c) The patient may have no symptoms or may complain of discomfort or a burning sensation at the tip of the tongue.

143 This patient has bilateral parotid gland enlargement due to sialosis.

144 (a) This tumour is clearly arising in the tonsillar region and is likely to be a non-Hodgkin's lymphoma.

(b) Non-Hodgkin's lymphoma can arise *de novo* but may also form part of the spectrum of diseases associated with HIV infection, as in this case.

(c) The prognosis for HIV-positive patients who develop non-Hodgkin's lymphoma is poor.

ANSWERS

145 (a) This young patient has white sponge naevus. It is an autosomal dominant condition inherited in a pattern of incomplete penetrance. In other words, both male and female offspring are affected but not always to the same degree. One or other parent must be affected by the condition to some extent.

(b) Surprisingly, systemic antibiotic therapy can be of some value in treating this condition. Clearly, in children tetracycline would be avoided but it would appear that even penicillin has some affect in reducing the extent of these lesions, by mechanisms that are unclear.

146 (a) This patient has lost filiform papilla on the left lateral aspect of the tongue, with some surrounding areas of hyperkeratosis. This is typical of geographic tongue.

(b) The microscopic features of geographic tongue are similar to psoriasis.

147 (a) This lesion was thought to be a denture-induced hyperplasia but clearly it is not because the overlying mucosa is not normal and is ulcerated in multiple areas.

(b) The likely diagnosis is squamous cell carcinoma, which in this patient was proven on biopsy.

148 (a) This patient has bilateral adherent plaques on the right and left lateral margins of the tongue. The condition is likely to be lichen planus.

(b) Management should involve biopsy to confirm the clinical diagnosis and, if the patient is asymptomatic, no treatment, but long-term review would be warranted. If the patient has symptoms then a variety of treatments, including topical steroids, may be used.

149 (a) This is angular cheilitis, in this case bilateral.

(b) The organisms that are usually responsible are *Candida* species or *Staphylococcus aureus*.

(b) In this patient, management would involve excluding haematinic deficiency states and a 7- or 14-day course of systemic fluconazole therapy.

150 If the patient complains of a burning sensation of the mouth, in the absence of any clinical abnormality, burning mouth syndrome is a possible diagnosis. Several variants of burning mouth syndrome are recognised and are termed type 1, type 2 and type 3. The clinical significance of these is important. In type 1 burning mouth syndrome the burning is present daily, is not present on waking but develops as the day progresses. In type 2 burning mouth syndrome the condition is present daily and is unchanged throughout the day. In type 3 burning mouth syndrome the condition is present on only some days. Certain features are common to all types of burning and in particular cases, such as type 3, investigations for allergy may be important. The 12 likely causes of burning sensation in the mouth are vitamin B_1 and B_6 deficiency, other haematinic deficiencies, such as iron and vitamin B_{12}, undiagnosed diabetes mellitus, candidal infection, a degree of xerostomia, cancer phobia, parafunctional activity, inappropriate denture design causing overloading of the mucosa, chronic anxiety and depression and allergy to a variety of substances.

151 (a) This patient has marked swelling in both the upper and lower lips, with a suggestion of angular cheilitis. The appearance is asymmetrical and typical of orofacial granulomatosis (OFG).

(b) OFG is not related to any bowel disease although clinically it mimics the oral manifestations of Crohn's disease.

(c) OFG is thought to be an allergic condition triggered by allergy to a variety of factors, including dyes, colourings, flavourings and preservatives.

INDEX

Numbers refer to the number shared by the illustration, question and answer.

Facial nerve palsy 53, 54, 72, 78
Fatty acids 67
Ferritin *see* Iron deficiency
Fibrin deposition 17
Fibromatosis 50, 139
Fibrous dysplasia 50
Fibrous epulis 13
Fibrous overgrowth
  dentures 16
  frictional irritation 88
  gingivae 3
  simple 42
Fine needle aspiration 12
Fluconazole 39, 43, 71, 76, 77, 111
Fluocinonide 14
Folic acid deficiency 83, 90
Fordyce spots 15
Foreign bodies 120
Frusemide 43

Gadolinium scans 62
Gardner's syndrome 134
Gastric ulcer 64
Geographic tongue (erythema migrans;
  benign migratory glossitis) 56, 88, 110,
  146
Giant cell granuloma, peripheral 36, 47
Giant cell lesions 13, 32, 36
Giant cell tumour 105
Giemsa stain 23
Gingivae
  biopsies 3, 13
  fibromatosis 50, 139
  fibrous overgrowth 3
  hyperplasia 32, 139
  pigmented lesions 56
  swelling 13, 36
Gingivitis, desquamative 14, 141
Gingivostomatitis, herpetic 96
Glandular fever 81
Glaucoma 8
Glossitis
  benign migratory (geographic tongue)
    56, 88, 110, 146
  medial rhomboid 121
Glue intoxication 75
Glyceryl trinitrate 65, 102
Gold therapy 18
Granulomas
  non-caseating epithelioid 82

peripheral giant cell 36, 47
pyogenic 3, 13, 32, 36, 47, 105, 120
Grinspan's syndrome 2
Griseofulvin 14, 49
Guillain–Barré syndrome 54

Haemangioma 51, 89
Haemophilia 95
Hairy leukoplakia 25, 93
Hamartoma 3, 140
Head and neck irradiation 40
Heck's disease 1
Hepatitis B 55, 95
Herpes labialis 9, 97
Herpes zoster infection 29
Herpetic gingivostomatitis 96
Herpetiform ulceration 66
Human immunodeficiency virus (HIV)
  infection 12, 21, 26, 38, 78, 90, 93, 144
Human papilloma virus 1, 25, 130
Hydrocortisone cream 3
Hydrocortisone hemisuccinate 47
Hypercementosis 50
Hypercholesterolaemia 67
Hyperkeratosis 10
Hyperparathyroidism 32
  brown tumour 36
Hyperpigmentation *see* Pigmentation
Hypersensitivity reactions, type-1 107
  see also Allergies
Hypertension, essential 2

Immunofluorescence 136
Infective endocarditis 91
Inflammatory bowel disease 119
Inhalers, steroid 121
In-situ hybridisation 1
Intraorbital nerve 29
Iron deficiency 7, 36, 77, 83, 90, 150
  anaemia 24, 119
Irradiation
  head and neck 40
  occupational exposure 98

Kaposi's sarcoma 12, 21
Kaposi's varicelliform eruption 96
Keratosis 88
  actinic 10
  smoker's 65, 77
  traumatic 77